JNANA YOGA

SWAMI VIVEKANANDA

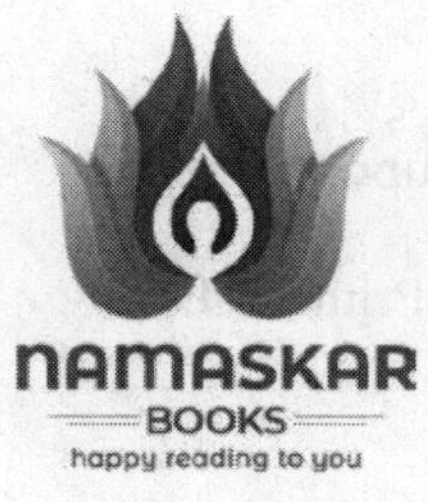

Published by
NAMASKAR BOOKS
Building No. 2/42 (Second Floor)
Ansari Road, Daryaganj
New Delhi-110002
e-mail: namaskarbooks@gmail.com
Website: www.namaskarbooks.com

ISBN: 978-93-5571-585-2

Jnana Yoga
By Swami Vivekanand

Edition 2026

Price
₹ 400.00 (Rupees Four Hundred only)

Printed at R-Tech Offset Printers, Delhi

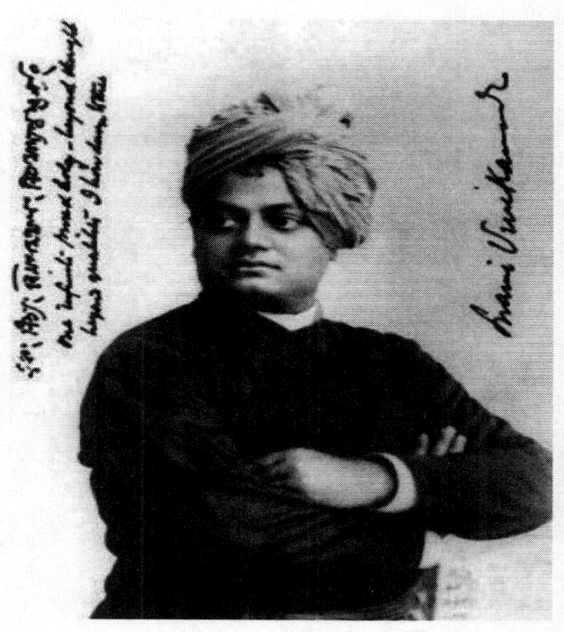

Based on lectures the Swami delivered in his rented rooms at 228 W 39th Street in December, 1895 and January, 1896. The classes were free of charge. Generally the Swami held two classes daily- morning and evening.

Although the Swami delivered many lectures and held numerous classes in the two years and five months he had been in America, these lectures constituted a departure in the way they were recorded. Just prior to the commencement of his Winter -95-96 season in NYC, his friends and supporters aided him by advertising for and ultimately hiring a professional stenographer: The man selected, Joseph Josiah Goodwin, later became a disciple of the Swami and followed him to England and India.

Four Paths of Yoga

(Written by the Swami during his first visit to America in answer to questions put by a Western disciple.)

Our main problem is to be free. It is evident then that until we realise ourselves as the Absolute, we cannot attain to deliverance. Yet there are various ways of attaining to this realisation. These methods have the generic name of Yoga (to join, to join ourselves to our reality). These Yogas, though divided into various groups, can principally be classed into four; and as each is only a method leading indirectly to the realisation of the Absolute, they are suited to different temperaments. Now it must be remembered that it is not that the assumed man becomes the real man or Absolute. There is no becoming with the Absolute. It is ever free, ever perfect; but the ignorance that has covered Its nature for a time is to be removed. Therefore the whole scope of all systems of Yoga (and each religion represents one) is to clear up this ignorance and allow the Âtman to restore its own nature. The chief helps in this liberation are Abhyâsa and Vairâgya. Vairagya is non-attachment to life, because it is the will to enjoy that brings all this bondage in its train; and Abhyasa is constant practice of any one of the Yogas.

Karma Yoga. Karma Yoga is purifying the mind by means of work. Now if any work is done, good or bad, it must produce as a result a good or bad effect; no power can stay it, once the cause is present. Therefore good action producing good Karma, and bad action, bad Karma, the soul will go on in eternal bondage without ever hoping for deliverance. Now Karma belongs only to the body or the mind, never to the Atman (Self); only it can cast a veil before the Atman. The veil cast by bad Karma is ignorance. Good Karma has the power to strengthen the moral powers. And thus it creates non-attachment; it destroys the tendency towards bad Karma and thereby purifies the mind. But if the work is done with the intention of enjoyment, it then produces only that very enjoyment and does not purify the mind or Chitta. Therefore all work should be done without any desire to enjoy the fruits thereof. All fear and all desire to enjoy here or hereafter must be banished for ever by the Karma-Yogi. Moreover, this Karma without desire of return will destroy the selfishness, which is the root of all bondage. The watchword of the Karma-Yogi is "not I, but Thou", and no amount of self-sacrifice is too much for him. But he does this without any desire to go to heaven, or gain name or fame or any other benefit in this world. Although the explanation and rationale of this unselfish work is only in Jnana Yoga, yet the natural divinity of man makes him love all sacrifice simply for the good of others, without any ulterior motive, whatever his creed or opinion. Again, with many the bondage of wealth is very great; and Karma Yoga is absolutely necessary for them as breaking the crystallisation that has gathered round their love of money.

Next is Bhakti Yoga. Bhakti or worship or love in some form or other is the easiest, pleasantest, and most natural way of man. The natural state of this universe is attraction; and that is surely followed by an ultimate disunion. Even so, love is the natural impetus of union in the human heart; and though itself a great cause of misery, properly directed towards the proper object, it brings deliverance. The object of Bhakti is God. Love cannot be without a subject and an object. The object of love again must be at first a being who can reciprocate our love. Therefore the God of love must be in some sense a human God. He must be a God of love. Aside from the question whether such a God exists or not, it is a fact that to those who have love in their heart this Absolute appears as a God of love, as personal.

The lower forms of worship, which embody the idea of God as a judge or punisher or someone to be obeyed through fear, do not deserve to be called love, although they are forms of worship gradually expanding into higher forms. We pass on to the consideration of love itself. We will illustrate love by a triangle, of which the first angle at the base is fearlessness. So long as there is fear, it is not love. Love banishes all fear. A mother with her baby will face a tiger to save her child. The second angle is that love never asks, never begs. The third or the apex is that love loves for the sake of love itself. Even the idea of object vanishes. Love is the only form in which love is loved. This is the highest abstraction and the same as the Absolute.

Next is Raja Yoga. This Yoga fits in with every one of these Yogas. It fits inquirers of all classes with or without any belief, and it is the real instrument of religious inquiry. As each science has its particular method of investigation, so is this Raja Yoga the method of religion. This science also is variously applied according to various constitutions. The chief parts are the Prânâyâma, concentration, and meditation. For those who believe in God, a symbolical name, such as Om or other sacred words received from a Guru, will be very helpful. Om is the greatest, meaning the Absolute. Meditating on the meaning of these holy names while repeating them is the chief practice.

Next is Jnana Yoga. This is divided into three parts. First: hearing the truth – that the Atman is the only reality and that everything else is Mâyâ (relativity). Second: reasoning upon this philosophy from all points of view. Third: giving up all further argumentation and realising the truth. This realisation comes from (1) being certain that Brahman is real and everything else is unreal; (2) giving up all desire for enjoyment; (3) controlling the senses and the mind; (4) intense desire to be free. Meditating on this reality always and reminding the soul of its real nature are the only ways in this Yoga. It is the highest, but most difficult. Many persons get an intellectual grasp of it, but very few attain realisation.

❑

Contents

1

The Necessity of Religion

(Delivered in London)

Of all the forces that have worked and are still working to mould the destinies of the human race, none, certainly, is more potent than that, the manifestation of which we call religion. All social organisations have as a background, somewhere, the workings of that peculiar force, and the greatest cohesive impulse ever brought into play amongst human units has been derived from this power. It is obvious to all of us that in very many cases the bonds of religion have proved stronger than the bonds of race, or climate, or even of descent. It is a well-known fact that persons worshipping the same God, believing in the same religion, have stood by each other, with much greater strength and constancy, than people of merely the same descent, or even brothers. Various attempts have been made to trace the beginnings of religion. In all the ancient religions which have come down to us at the present day, we find one claim made — that they are all supernatural, that their genesis is not, as it were, in the human brain, but that they have originated somewhere outside of it.

Two theories have gained some acceptance amongst modern scholars. One is the spirit theory of religion, the other the evolution of the idea of the Infinite. One party maintains that ancestor worship is the beginning of religious ideas; the other, that religion originates in the personification of the powers of nature. Man wants to keep up the memory of his dead relatives and thinks they are living even when the body is dissolved, and he wants to place food for them and, in a certain sense, to worship them. Out of that came the growth we call religion.

Studying the ancient religions of the Egyptians, Babylonians, Chinese, and many other races in America and elsewhere, we find very clear traces of this ancestor worship being the beginning of religion. With the ancient Egyptians, the first idea of the soul was that of a double. Every human body contained in it another being very similar to it; and when a man died, this double went out of the body and yet lived on. But the life of the double lasted only so long as the dead body remained intact, and that is why we find among the Egyptians so much solicitude to keep the body uninjured. And that is why they built those huge pyramids in which they preserved the bodies. For, if any portion of the external body was hurt, the double would be correspondingly injured. This is clearly ancestor worship. With the ancient Babylonians we find the same idea of the double, but with a variation. The double lost all sense of love; it frightened the living to give it food and drink, and to help it in various ways. It even lost all affection for its own children and its own wife. Among the ancient Hindus also, we find traces of this ancestor worship. Among the Chinese, the basis of their religion may also be said to be ancestor worship, and it still permeates the length and breadth of that vast country. In fact, the only religion that can really be said to flourish in China is that of ancestor worship. Thus it seems, on the one hand, a very good position is made out for those who hold the theory of ancestor worship as the beginning of religion.

On the other hand, there are scholars who from the ancient Aryan literature show that religion originated in nature worship. Although in India we find proofs of ancestor worship everywhere, yet in the oldest records there is no trace of it whatsoever. In the Rig-Veda Samhitâ, the most ancient record of the Aryan race, we do not find any trace of it. Modern scholars think, it is the worship of nature that they find there. The human mind seems to struggle to get a peep behind the scenes. The dawn, the evening, the hurricane, the stupendous and gigantic forces of nature, its beauties, these have exercised the human mind, and it aspires to go beyond, to understand something about them. In the struggle they endow these phenomena with personal attributes, giving them souls and bodies, sometimes beautiful, sometimes transcendent. Every attempt ends by these phenomena becoming abstractions whether personalised or not. So also it is found with the ancient Greeks; their whole mythology is simply this abstracted nature worship. So also with the ancient Germans, the Scandinavians, and all the other Aryan races. Thus, on this side, too, a very strong case has been made out, that religion has its origin in the personification of the powers of nature.

These two views, though they seem to be contradictory, can be reconciled on a third basis, which, to my mind, is the real germ of religion, and that I propose to call the struggle to transcend the limitations of the senses. Either, man goes to seek for the spirits of his ancestors, the spirits of the dead, that is, he wants to get a glimpse of what there is after the body is dissolved, or, he desires to understand the power working behind the stupendous phenomena of nature. Whichever of these is the case, one thing is certain, that he tries to transcend the limitations of the senses. He cannot remain satisfied with his senses; he wants to go beyond them. The explanation need not be mysterious. To me it seems very natural that the first glimpse of religion should come through dreams. The first idea of immortality man may well get through dreams. Is that not a most wonderful state? And we know that children and untutored minds find very little difference between dreaming and their awakened state. What can be more natural than that they find, as natural logic, that even during the sleep state when the body is apparently dead, the mind goes on with all its intricate workings? What wonder that men will at once come to the conclusion that when this body is dissolved for ever, the same working will go on? This, to my mind, would be a more natural explanation of the supernatural, and through this dream idea the human mind rises to higher and higher conceptions. Of course, in time, the vast majority of mankind found out that these dreams are not verified by their waking states, and that during the dream state it is not that man has a fresh existence, but simply that he recapitulates the experiences of the awakened state.

But by this time the search had begun, and the search was inward, arid man continued inquiring more deeply into the different stages of the mind and discovered higher states than either the waking or the dreaming. This state of things we find in all the organised religions of the world, called either ecstasy or inspiration. In all organised religions, their founders, prophets, and messengers are declared to have gone into states of mind that were neither waking nor sleeping, in which they came face to face with a new series of facts relating to what is called the spiritual kingdom. They realised things there much more intensely than we realise facts around us in our waking state. Take, for instance, the religions of the Brahmins. The Vedas are said to be written by Rishis. These Rishis were sages who realised certain facts. The exact definition of the Sanskrit word Rishi is a Seer of Mantras – of the thoughts conveyed in the Vedic hymns. These men declared that they had realised – sensed, if that word can be used with regard to the supersensuous – certain facts, and these facts they proceeded to put on record. We find the same truth declared amongst both the Jews and the Christians.

Some exceptions may be taken in the case of the Buddhists as represented by the Southern sect. It may be asked – if the Buddhists do not believe in any God or soul, how can their religion be derived from the supersensuous state of existence? The answer to this is that even the Buddhists find an eternal moral law, and that moral law was not reasoned out in our sense of the word But Buddha found it, discovered it, in a supersensuous state. Those of you who have studied the life of Buddha even as briefly given in that beautiful poem, *The Light of Asia*, may remember that Buddha is represented as sitting under the Bo-tree until he reached that supersensuous state of mind. All his teachings came through this, and not through intellectual cogitations.

Thus, a tremendous statement is made by all religions; that the human mind, at certain moments, transcends not only the limitations of the senses, but also the power of reasoning. It then comes face to face with facts which it could never have sensed, could never hive reasoned out. These facts are the basis of all the religions of the world. Of course we have the right to challenge these facts, to put them to the test of reason. Nevertheless, all the existing religions of the world claim for the human mind this peculiar power of transcending the limits of the senses and the limits of reason; and this power they put forward as a statement of fact.

Apart from the consideration of tie question how far these facts claimed by religions are true, we find one characteristic common to them all. They are all abstractions as contrasted with the concrete discoveries of physics, for instance; and in all the highly organised religions they take the purest form of Unit Abstraction, either in the form of an Abstracted Presence, as an Omnipresent Being, as an Abstract Personality called God, as a Moral Law, or in the form of an Abstract Essence underlying every existence. In modern times, too, the attempts made to preach religions without appealing to the supersensuous state if the mind have had to take up the old abstractions of the Ancients and give different names to them as "Moral Law", the "Ideal Unity", and so forth, thus showing that these abstractions are not in the senses. None of us have yet seen an "Ideal Human Being", and yet we are told to believe in it. None of us have yet seen an ideally perfect man, and yet without that ideal we cannot progress. Thus, this one fact stands out from all these different religions, that there is an Ideal Unit Abstraction, which is put before us, either in the form of a Person or an Impersonal Being, or a Law, or a Presence, or an Essence. We are always struggling to raise ourselves up to that ideal. Every human being, whosoever and wheresoever he may be, has an ideal of infinite power. Every human being has an ideal of infinite pleasure. Most of the works that we find around us, the activities displayed everywhere, are due to the struggle for this infinite power or this infinite pleasure. But a few quickly discover that although they are struggling for infinite power, it is not through the senses that it can be reached. They find out very soon that that infinite pleasure is not to be got through the senses, or, in other words, the senses are too limited, and the body is too limited, to express the Infinite. To manifest the Infinite through the finite is impossible, and sooner or later, man learns to give up the attempt to express the Infinite through the finite. This giving up, this renunciation of the attempt, is the background of ethics. Renunciation is the very basis upon which ethics stands. There never was an ethical code preached which had not renunciation for its basis.

Ethics always says, "Not I, but thou." Its motto is, "Not self, but non-self." The vain ideas of individualism, to which man clings when he is trying to find that Infinite Power or that Infinite Pleasure through the senses, have to be given up — say the laws of ethics. You have to put *yourself* last, and others before you. The senses say, "Myself first." Ethics says, "I must hold myself last." Thus, all codes of ethics are based upon this renunciation; destruction, not construction, of the individual on the material plane. That Infinite will never find expression upon the material plane, nor is it possible or thinkable.

So, man has to give up the plane of matter and rise to other spheres to seek a deeper expression of that Infinite. In this way the various ethical laws are being moulded, but all have that one central idea, eternal self-abnegation. Perfect self-annihilation is the ideal of ethics. People are startled if they are asked not to think of their individualities. They seem so very much afraid of losing what they call their individuality. At the same time, the same men would declare the highest ideals of ethics to be right, never for a moment thinking that the scope, the goal, the idea of all ethics is the destruction, and not the building up, of the individual.

Utilitarian standards cannot explain the ethical relations of men, for, in the first place, we cannot derive any ethical laws from considerations of utility. Without the supernatural sanction as it is called, or the perception of the superconscious as I prefer to term it, there can be no ethics. Without the struggle towards the Infinite there can be no ideal. Any system that wants to bind men down to the limits of their own societies is not able to find an explanation for the ethical laws of mankind. The Utilitarian wants us to give up the struggle after the Infinite, the reaching-out for the Supersensuous, as impracticable and absurd, and, in the same breath, asks us to take up ethics and do good to society. Why should we do good?

Doing good is a secondary consideration. We must have an ideal. Ethics itself is not the end, but the means to the end. If the end is not there, why should we be ethical? Why should I do good to other men, and not injure them? If happiness is the goal of mankind, why should I not make myself happy and others unhappy? What prevents me? In the second place, the basis of utility is too narrow. All the current social forms and methods are derived from society as it exists, but what right has the Utilitarian to assume that society is eternal? Society did not exist ages ago, possibly will not exist ages hence. Most probably it is one of the passing stages through which we are going towards a higher evolution, and any law that is derived from society alone cannot be eternal, cannot cover the whole ground of man's nature. At best, therefore, Utilitarian theories can only work under present social conditions. Beyond that they have no value. But a morality an ethical code, derived from religion and spirituality, has the whole of infinite man for its scope. It takes up the individual, but its relations are to the Infinite, and it takes up society also – because society is nothing but numbers of these individuals grouped together; and as it applies to the individual and *his* eternal relations, it must necessarily apply to the whole of society, in whatever condition it may be at any given time. Thus we see that there is always the necessity of spiritual religion for mankind. Man cannot always think of matter, however pleasurable it may be.

It has been said that too much attention to things spiritual disturbs our practical relations in this world. As far back as in the days of the Chinese sage Confucius, it was said, "Let us take care of this world: and then, when we have finished with this world, we will take care of other world." It is very well that we should *take care* of this world. But if too much attention to the spiritual may affect a little our practical relations, too much attention to the so-called practical hurts us here and hereafter. It makes us materialistic. For man is not to regard *nature* as his goal, but something higher.

Man is man so long as he is struggling to rise above nature, and this nature is both internal and external. Not only does it comprise the laws that govern the particles of matter outside us and in our bodies, but also the more subtle nature within, which is, in fact, the motive power governing the external. It is good and very grand to conquer external nature, but grander still to conquer our internal nature. It is grand and good to know the laws that govern the stars and planets; it is infinitely grander and better to know the laws that govern the passions, the feelings, the will, of mankind. This conquering of the inner man, understanding the secrets of the subtle workings that are within the human mind, and knowing its wonderful secrets, belong entirely to religion. Human nature – the ordinary human nature, I mean – wants to see big material facts. The ordinary man cannot understand anything that is subtle. Well has it been said that the masses admire the lion that kills a thousand lambs, never for a moment thinking that it is death to the lambs. Although a momentary triumph for the lion; because they find pleasure only in manifestations of physical strength. Thus it is with the ordinary run of mankind. They understand and find pleasure in everything that is external. But in every society there is a section whose pleasures are not in the senses, but beyond, and who now and then catch glimpses of something higher than matter and struggle to reach it. And if we read the history of nations between the lines, we shall always find that the rise of a nation comes with an increase in the number of such men; and the fall begins when this pursuit after the Infinite, however vain Utilitarians may call it, has ceased. That is to say, the mainspring of the strength Of every race lies in its spirituality, and the death of that race begins the day that spirituality wanes and materialism gains ground.

Thus, apart from the solid facts and truths that we may learn from religion, apart from the comforts that we may gain from it, religion, as a science, as a study, is the greatest and healthiest exercise that the human mind can have. This pursuit of the Infinite, this struggle to grasp the Infinite, this effort to get beyond the limitations of the senses – out of matter, as it were – and to evolve the spiritual man – this striving day and night to make the Infinite one with our being – this struggle itself is the grandest and most glorious that man can make. Some persons find the greatest pleasure in eating. We have no right to say that they should not. Others find the greatest pleasure in possessing certain things. We have no right to say that they should not. But they also have no right to say "no" to the man who finds his highest pleasure in spiritual thought. The lower the organisation, the greater the pleasure in the senses. Very few men can eat a meal with the same gusto as a dog or a wolf. But all the pleasures of the dog or the wolf have gone, as it were into the senses. The lower types of humanity in all nations find pleasure in the senses, while the cultured and the educated find it in thought, in philosophy, in arts and sciences. Spirituality is a still higher plane. The subject being infinite, that plane is the highest, and the pleasure there is the highest for those who can appreciate it. So, even on the utilitarian ground that man is to seek for pleasure, he should cultivate religious thought, for it is the highest pleasure that exists. Thus religion, as a study, seems to me to be absolutely necessary.

We can see it in its effects. It is the greatest motive power that moves the human mind No other ideal can put into us the same mass of energy as the spiritual. So far as human history goes, it is obvious to all of us that this has been the case and that its powers are not dead. I do not deny that men, on simply utilitarian grounds, can be very good and moral. There have been many great men in this world perfectly sound, moral, and good, simply on utilitarian grounds. But the world-movers, men who bring, as It were, a mass of magnetism into the world whose spirit works in hundreds and in thousands, whose life ignites others with a spiritual fire — such men, we always find, have that spiritual background. Their motive power came from religion. Religion is the greatest motive power for realising that infinite energy which is the birthright and nature of every man. In building up character in making for everything that is good and great, in bringing peace to others and peace to one's own self, religion is the highest motive power and, therefore, ought to be studied from that standpoint. Religion must be studied on a broader basis than formerly. All narrow limited, fighting ideas of religion have to go. All sect ideas and tribal or national ideas of religion must be given up. That each tribe or nation should have its own particular God and think that every other is wrong is a superstition that should belong to the past. All such ideas must be abandoned.

As the human mind broadens, its spiritual steps broaden too. The time has already come when a man cannot record a thought without its reaching to all corners of the earth; by merely physical means, we have come into touch with the whole world; so the future religions of the world have to become as universal, as wide.

The religious ideals of the future must embrace all that exists in the world and is good and great, and, at the same time, have infinite scope for future development. All that was good in the past must be preserved; and the doors must be kept open for future additions to the already existing store. Religions must also be inclusive and not look down with contempt upon one another because their particular ideals of God are different. In my life I have seen a great many spiritual men, a great many sensible persons, who did not believe in God at all that is to say, not in our sense of the word. Perhaps they understood God better than we can ever do. The Personal idea of God or the Impersonal, the Infinite, Moral Law, or the Ideal Man — these all have to come under the definition of religion. And when religions have become thus broadened, their power for good will have increased a hundredfold. Religions, having tremendous power in them, have often done more injury to the world than good, simply on account of their narrowness and limitations.

Even at the present time we find many sects and societies, with almost the same ideas, fighting each other, because one does not want to set forth those ideas in precisely the same way as another. Therefore, religions will have to broaden. Religious ideas will have to become universal, vast, and infinite; and then alone we shall have the fullest play of religion, for the power of religion has only just begun to manifest in the world. It is sometimes said that religions are dying out, that spiritual ideas are dying out of the world. To me it seems that they have just begun to grow. The power of religion, broadened and purified, is going to penetrate every part of human life. So long as religion was in the hands of a chosen few or of a body of priests, it was in temples, churches, books, dogmas, ceremonials, forms, and rituals. But when we come to the real, spiritual, universal concept, then, and then alone religion will become real and living; it will come into our very nature, live in our every movement, penetrate every pore of our society, and be infinitely more a power for good than it has ever been before.

What is needed is a fellow-feeling between the different types of religion, seeing that they all stand or fall together, a fellow-feeling which springs from mutual esteem and mutual respect, and not the condescending, patronising, niggardly expression of goodwill, unfortunately in vogue at the present time with many. And above all, this is needed between types of religious expression coming from the study of mental phenomena — unfortunately, even now laying exclusive claim to the name of religion — and those expressions of religion whose heads, as it were, are penetrating more into the secrets of heaven though their feet are clinging to earth, I mean the so-called materialistic sciences.

To bring about this harmony, both will have to make concessions, sometimes very large, nay more, sometimes painful, but each will find itself the better for the sacrifice and more advanced in truth. And in the end, the knowledge which is confined within the domain of time and space will meet and become one with that which is beyond them both, where the mind and senses cannot reach — the Absolute, the Infinite, the One without a second.

❑

2

The Real Nature of Man

(*Delivered in London*)

Great is the tenacity with which man clings to the senses. Yet, however substantial he may think the external world in which he lives and moves, there comes a time in the lives of individuals and of races when, involuntarily, they ask, "Is this real?" To the person who never finds a moment to question the credentials of his senses, whose every moment is occupied with some sort of sense-enjoyment – even to him death comes, and he also is compelled to ask, "Is this real?" Religion begins with this question and ends with its answer. Even in the remote past, where recorded history cannot help us, in the mysterious light of mythology, back in the dim twilight of civilisation, we find the same question was asked, "What becomes of this? What is real?"

One of the most poetical of the Upanishads, the Katha Upanishad, begins with the inquiry: "When a man dies, there is a dispute. One party declares that he has gone for ever, the other insists that he is still living. Which is true?" Various answers have been given. The whole sphere of metaphysics, philosophy, and religion is really filled with various answers to this question. At the same time, attempts have been made to suppress it, to put a stop to the unrest of mind which asks, "What is beyond? What is real?" But so long as death remains, all these attempts at suppression will always prove to be unsuccessful. We may talk about seeing nothing beyond and keeping all our hopes and aspirations confined to the present moment, and struggle hard not to think of anything beyond the world of senses; and, perhaps, everything outside helps to keep us limited within its narrow bounds. The whole world may combine to prevent us from broadening out beyond the present. Yet, so long as there is death, the question must come again and again, "Is death the end of all these things to which we are clinging, as if they were the most real of all realities, the most substantial of all substances?" The world vanishes in a moment and is gone. Standing on the brink of a precipice beyond which is the infinite yawning chasm, every mind, however hardened, is bound to recoil and ask, "Is this real?" The hopes of a lifetime, built up little by little with all the energies of a great mind, vanish in a second. Are they real? This question must be answered. Time never lessens its power; on the other hand, it adds strength to it.

Then there is the desire to be happy. We run after everything to make ourselves happy; we pursue our mad career in the external world of senses. If you ask the young man with whom life is successful, he will declare that it is real; and he really thinks so. Perhaps, when the same man grows old and finds fortune ever eluding him, he will then declare that it is fate. He finds at last that his desires cannot be fulfilled. Wherever he goes, there is an adamantine wall beyond which he cannot pass. Every sense-activity results in a reaction. Everything is evanescent. Enjoyment, misery, luxury, wealth, power, and poverty, even life itself, are all evanescent.

Two positions remain to mankind. One is to believe with the nihilists that all is nothing, that we know nothing, that we can never know anything either about the future, the past, or even the present. For we must remember that he who denies the past and the future and wants to stick to the present is simply a madman. One may as well deny the father and mother and assert the child. It would be equally logical. To deny the past and future, the present must inevitably be denied also. This is one position, that of the nihilists. I have never seen a man who could really become a nihilist for one minute. It is very easy to talk.

Then there is the other position — to seek for an explanation, to seek for the real, to discover in the midst of this eternally changing and evanescent world whatever is real. In this body which is an aggregate of molecules of matter, is there anything which is real? This has been the search throughout the history of the, human mind. In the very oldest times, we often find glimpses of light coming into men's minds. We find man, even then, going a step beyond this body, finding something which is not this external body, although very much like it, much more complete, much more perfect, and which remains even when this body is dissolved. We read in the hymns of the Rig-Veda, addressed to the God of Fire who is burning a dead body, "Carry him, O Fire, in your arms gently, give him a perfect body, a bright body, carry him where the fathers live, where there is no more sorrow, where there is no more death." The same idea you will find present in every religion. And we get another idea with it. It is a significant fact that all religions, without one exception, hold that man is a degeneration of what he was, whether they clothe this in mythological words, or in the clear language of philosophy, or in the beautiful expressions of poetry. This is the one fact that comes out of every scripture and of every mythology that the man that is, is a degeneration of what he was. This is the kernel of truth within the story of Adam's fall in the Jewish scripture. This is again and again repeated in the scriptures of the Hindus; the dream of a period which they call the Age of Truth, when no man died unless he wished to die, when he could keep his body as long as he liked, and his mind was pure and strong. There was no evil and no misery; and the present age is a corruption of that state of perfection. Side by side with this, we find the story of the deluge everywhere. That story itself is a proof that this present age is held to be a corruption of a former age by every religion. It went on becoming more and more corrupt until the deluge swept away a large portion of mankind, and again the ascending series began. It is going up slowly again to reach once more that early state of purity. You are all aware of the story of the deluge in the Old Testament. The same story was current among the ancient Babylonians, the Egyptians, the Chinese, and the Hindus. Manu, a great ancient sage, was praying on the bank of the Gangâ, when a little minnow came to him for protection, and he put it into a pot of water he had before him. "What do you want?" asked Manu. The little minnow declared he was pursued by a bigger fish and wanted protection. Manu carried the little fish to his home, and in the morning he had become as big as the pot and said, "I cannot live in this pot any longer". Manu put him in a tank, and the next day he was as big as the tank and declared he could not live there any more. So Manu had to take him to a river, and in the morning the fish filled the river. Then Manu put him in the ocean, and he declared, "Manu, I am the Creator of the universe. I have taken this form to come and warn you that I will deluge the world. You build an ark and in it put a pair of every kind of animal, and let your family enter the ark, and there will project out of the water my horn. Fasten the ark to it; and when the deluge subsides, come out and people the earth." So the world was deluged, and Manu saved his own family and two of every kind of animal and seeds of every plant. When the deluge subsided, he came and peopled the world; and we are all called "man", because we are the progeny of Manu.

Now, human language is the attempt to express the truth that is within. I am fully persuaded that a baby whose language consists of unintelligible sounds is attempting to express the highest philosophy, only the baby has not the organs to express it nor the means. The difference between the language of the highest philosophers and the utterances of babies is one of degree and not of kind. What you call the most correct, systematic, mathematical language of the present time, and the hazy, mystical, mythological languages of the ancients, differ only in degree. All of them have a grand idea behind, which is, as it were, struggling to express itself; and often behind these ancient mythologies are nuggets of truth; and often, I am sorry to say, behind the fine, polished phrases of the moderns is arrant trash. So, we need not throw a thing overboard because it is clothed in mythology, because it does not fit in with the notions of Mr. So-and-so or Mrs. So-and-so of modern times. If people should laugh at religion because most religions declare that men must believe in mythologies taught by such and such a prophet, they ought to laugh more at these moderns. In modern times, if a man quotes a Moses or a Buddha or a Christ, he is laughed at; but let him give the name of a Huxley, a Tyndall, or a Darwin, and it is swallowed without salt. "Huxley has said it", that is enough for many. We are free from superstitions indeed! That was a religious superstition, and this a scientific superstition; only, in and through that superstition came life-giving ideas of spirituality; in and through this modern superstition come lust and greed. That superstition was worship of God, and this superstition is worship of filthy lucre, of fame or power. That is the difference.

To return to mythology. Behind all these stories we find one idea standing supreme – that man is a degeneration of what he was. Coming to the present times, modern research seems to repudiate this position absolutely. Evolutionists seem to contradict entirely this assertion. According to them, man is the evolution of the mollusc; and, therefore, what mythology states cannot be true. There is in India, however, a mythology which is able to reconcile both these positions. The Indian mythology has a theory of cycles, that all progression is in the form of waves. Every wave is attended by a fall, and that by a rise the next moment, that by a fall in the next, and again another rise The motion is in cycles. Certainly it is true, even on the grounds of modern research, that man cannot be simply an evolution. Every evolution presupposes an involution. The modern scientific man will tell you that you can only get the amount of energy out of a machine which you have previously put into it. Something cannot be produced out of nothing. If a man is an evolution of the mollusc, then the perfect man – the Buddha-man, the Christ-man – was involved in the mollusc. If it is not so, whence come these gigantic personalities? Something cannot come out of nothing. Thus we are in the position of reconciling the scriptures with modern light. That energy which manifests itself slowly through various stages until it becomes the perfect man, cannot come out of nothing. It existed somewhere; and if the mollusc or the protoplasm is the first point to which you can trace it, that protoplasm, somehow or other, must have contained the energy.

There is a great discussion going on as to whether the aggregate of materials we call the body is the cause of manifestation of the force we call the soul, thought, etc., or whether it is the thought that manifests this body. The religions of the world of course hold that the force called thought manifests the body, and not the reverse. There are schools of modern thought which hold that what we call thought is simply the outcome of the adjustment of the parts of the machine which we call body. Taking the second position that the soul or the mass of thought, or however you may call it, is the outcome of this machine, the outcome of the chemical and physical combinations of matter making up the body and brain, leaves the question unanswered. What makes the body? What force combines the molecules into the body form? What force is there which takes up material from the mass of matter around and forms my body one way, another body another way, and so on? What makes these infinite distinctions? To say that the force called soul is the outcome of the combinations of the molecules of the body is putting the cart before the horse. How did the combinations come; where was the force to make them? If you say that some other force was the cause of these combinations, and soul was the outcome of that matter, and that soul – which combined a certain mass of matter – was itself the result of the combinations, it is no answer. That theory ought to be taken which explains most of the facts, if not all, and that without contradicting other existing theories. It is more logical to say that the force which takes up the matter and forms the body is the same which manifests through that body. To say, therefore, that the thought forces manifested by the body are the outcome of the arrangement of molecules and have no independent existence has no meaning; neither can force evolve out of matter. Rather it is possible to demonstrate that what we call matter does not exist at all. It is only a certain state of force. Solidity, hardness, or any other state of matter can be proved to be the result of motion. Increase of vortex motion imparted to fluids gives them the force of solids. A mass of air in vortex motion, as in a tornado, becomes solid-like and by its impact breaks or cuts through solids. A thread of a spider's web, if it could be moved at almost infinite velocity, would be as strong as an iron chain and would cut through an oak tree. Looking at it in this way, it would be easier to prove that what we call matter does not exist. But the other way cannot be proved.

What is the force which manifests itself through the body? It is obvious to all of us, whatever that force be, that it is taking particles up, as it were, and manipulating forms out of them – the human body. None else comes here to manipulate bodies for you and me. I never saw anybody eat food for me. I have to assimilate it, manufacture blood and bones and everything out of that food. What is this mysterious force? Ideas about the future and about the past seem to be terrifying to many. To many they seem to be mere speculation.

We will take the present theme. What is this force which is now working through us? We know how in old times, in all the ancient scriptures, this power, this manifestation of power, was thought to be a bright substance having the form of this body, and which remained even after this body fell. Later on, however, we find a higher idea coming – that this bright body did not represent the force. Whatsoever has form must be the result of combinations of particles and requires something else behind it to move it. If this body requires something which is not the body to manipulate it, the bright body, by the same necessity, will also require something other than itself to manipulate it. So, that something was called the soul, the Atman in Sanskrit. It was the Atman which through the bright body, as it were, worked on the gross body outside. The bright body is considered as the receptacle of the mind, and the Atman is beyond that It is not the mind even; it works the mind, and through the mind the body. You have an Atman, I have another each one of us has a separate Atman and a separate fine body, and through that we work on the gross external body. Questions were then asked about this Atman about its nature. What is this Atman, this soul of man which is neither the body nor the mind? Great discussions followed. Speculations were made, various shades of philosophic inquiry came into existence; and I shall try to place before you some of the conclusions that have been reached about this Atman.

The different philosophies seem to agree that this Atman, whatever it be, has neither form nor shape, and that which has neither form nor shape must be omnipresent. Time begins with mind, space also is in the mind. Causation cannot stand without time. Without the idea of succession there cannot be any idea of causation. Time, space and causation, therefore, are in the mind, and as this Atman is beyond the mind and formless, it must be beyond time, beyond space, and beyond causation. Now, if it is beyond time, space, and causation, it must be infinite. Then comes the highest speculation in our philosophy. The infinite cannot be two. If the soul be infinite, there can be only one Soul, and all ideas of various souls — you having one soul, and I having another, and so forth — are not real. The Real Man, therefore, is one and infinite, the omnipresent Spirit. And the apparent man is only a limitation of that Real Man. In that sense the mythologies are true that the apparent man, however great he may be, is only a dim reflection of the Real Man who is beyond. The Real Man, the Spirit, being beyond cause and effect, not bound by time and space, must, therefore, be free. He was never bound, and could not be bound. The apparent man, the reflection, is limited by time, space, and causation, and is, therefore, bound. Or in the language of some of our philosophers, he appears to be bound, but really is not. This is the reality in our souls, this omnipresence, this spiritual nature, this infinity. Every soul is infinite, therefore there is no question of birth and death. Some children were being examined. The examiner put them rather hard questions, and among them was this one: "Why does not the earth fall?" He wanted to evoke answers about gravitation. Most of the children could not answer at all; a few answered that it was gravitation or something. One bright little girl answered it by putting another question: "Where should it fall?" The question is nonsense. Where should the earth fall? There is no falling or rising for the earth. In infinite space there is no up or down; that is only in the relative. Where is the going or coming for the infinite? Whence should it come and whither should it go?

Thus, when people cease to think of the past or future, when they give up the idea of body, because the body comes and goes and is limited, then they have risen to a higher ideal. The body is not the Real Man, neither is the mind, for the mind waxes and wanes. It is the Spirit beyond, which alone can live for ever. The body and mind are continually changing, and are, in fact, only names of series of changeful phenomena, like rivers whose waters are in a constant state of flux, yet presenting the appearance of unbroken streams. Every particle in this body is continually changing; no one has the same body for many minutes together, and yet we think of it as the same body. So with the mind; one moment it is happy, another moment unhappy; one moment strong, another weak; an ever-changing whirlpool. That cannot be the Spirit which is infinite. Change can only be in the limited. To say that the infinite changes in any way is absurd; it cannot be. You can move and I can move, as limited bodies; every particle in this universe is in a constant state of flux, but taking the universe as a unit, as one whole, it cannot move, it cannot change. Motion is always a relative thing. I move in relation to something else. Any particle in this universe can change in relation to any other particle; but take the whole universe as one, and in relation to what can it move? There is nothing besides it. So this infinite Unit is unchangeable, immovable, absolute, and this is the Real Man. Our reality, therefore, consists in the Universal and not in the limited. These are old delusions, however comfortable they are, to think that we are little limited beings, constantly changing. People are frightened when they are told that they are Universal Being, everywhere present. Through everything you work, through every foot you move, through every lip you talk, through every heart you feel.

People are frightened when they are told this. They will again and again ask you if they are not going to keep their individuality. What is individuality? I should like to see it. A baby has no moustache; when he grows to be a man, perhaps he has a moustache and beard. His individuality would be lost, if it were in the body. If I lose one eye, or if I lose one of my hands, my individuality would be lost if it were in the body. Then, a drunkard should not give up drinking because he would lose his individuality. A thief should not be a good man because he would thereby lose his individuality. No man ought to change his habits for fear of this. There is no individuality except in the Infinite. That is the only condition which does not change. Everything else is in a constant state of flux. Neither can individuality be in memory. Suppose, on account of a blow on the head I forget all about my past; then, I have lost all individuality; I am gone. I do not remember two or three years of my childhood, and if memory and existence are one, then whatever I forget is gone. That part of my life which I do not remember, I did not live. That is a very narrow idea of individuality.

We are not individuals yet. We are struggling towards individuality, and that is the Infinite, that is the real nature of man. He alone lives whose life is in the whole universe, and the more we concentrate our lives on limited things, the faster we go towards death. Those moments alone we live when our lives are in the universe, in others; and living this little life is death, simply death, and that is why the fear of death comes. The fear of death can only be conquered when man realises that so long as there is one life in this universe, he is living. When he can say, "I am in everything, in everybody, I am in all lives, I am the universe," then alone comes the state of fearlessness. To talk of immortality in constantly changing things is absurd. Says an old Sanskrit philosopher: It is only the Spirit that is the individual, because it is infinite. No infinity can be divided; infinity cannot be broken into pieces. It is the same one, undivided unit for ever, and this is the individual man, the Real Man. The apparent man is merely a struggle to express, to manifest this individuality which is beyond; and evolution is not in the Spirit. These changes which are going on — the wicked becoming good, the animal becoming man, take them in whatever way you like — are not in the Spirit. They are evolution of nature and manifestation of Spirit. Suppose there is a screen hiding you from me, in which there is a small hole through which I can see some of the faces before me, just a few faces. Now suppose the hole begins to grow larger and larger, and as it does so, more and more of the scene before me reveals itself and when at last the whole screen has disappeared, I stand face to face with you all. You did not change at all in this case; it was the hole that was evolving, and you were gradually manifesting yourselves. So it is with the Spirit. No perfection is going to be attained. You are already free and perfect. What are these ideas of religion and God and searching for the hereafter? Why does man look for a God? Why does man, in every nation, in every state of society, want a perfect ideal somewhere, either in man, in God, or elsewhere? Because that idea is within you. It was your own heart beating and you did not know; you were mistaking it for something external. It is the God within your own self that is propelling you to seek for Him, to realise Him. After long searches here and there, in temples and in churches, in earths and in heavens, at last you come back, completing the circle from where you started, to your own soul and find that He for whom you have been seeking all over the world, for whom you have been weeping and praying in churches and temples, on whom you were looking as the mystery of all mysteries shrouded in the clouds, is nearest of the near, is your own Self, the reality of your life, body, and soul. That is your own nature. Assert it, manifest it. Not to become pure, you are pure already. You are not to be perfect, you are that already. Nature is like that screen which is hiding the reality beyond. Every good thought that you think or act upon is simply tearing the veil, as it were; and the purity, the Infinity, the God behind, manifests Itself more and more.

This is the whole history of man. Finer and finer becomes the veil, more and more of the light behind shines forth, for it is its nature to shine. It cannot be known; in vain we try to know it. Were it knowable, it would not be what it is, for it is the eternal subject. Knowledge is a limitation, knowledge is objectifying. He is the eternal subject of everything, the eternal witness in this universe, your own Self. Knowledge is, as it were, a lower step, a degeneration. We are that eternal subject already; how can we know it? It is the real nature of every man, and he is struggling to express it in various ways; otherwise, why are there so many ethical codes? Where is the explanation of all ethics? One idea stands out as the centre of all ethical systems, expressed in various forms, namely, doing good to others. The guiding motive of mankind should be charity towards men, charity towards all animals. But these are all various expressions of that eternal truth that, "I am the universe; this universe is one." Or else, where is the reason? Why should I do good to my fellowmen? Why should I do good to others? What compels me? It is sympathy, the feeling of sameness everywhere. The hardest hearts feel sympathy for other beings sometimes. Even the man who gets frightened if he is told that this assumed individuality is really a delusion, that it is ignoble to try to cling to this apparent individuality, that very man will tell you that extreme self-abnegation is the centre of all morality. And what is perfect self-abnegation? It means the abnegation of this apparent self, the abnegation of all selfishness. This idea of "me and mine" — Ahamkâra and Mamatâ — is the result of past Superstition, and the more this present self passes away, the more the real Self becomes manifest. This is true self-abnegation, the centre, the basis, the gist of all moral teaching; and whether man knows it or not the whole world is slowly going towards it, practicing it more or less. Only, the vast majority of mankind are doing it unconsciously. Let them do it consciously. Let then make the sacrifice, knowing that this "me and mine" is not the real Self, but only a limitation. But one glimpse Of that infinite reality which is behind — but one spark of that infinite fire that is the All — represents the present man; the Infinite is his true nature.

What is the utility, the effect, the result, of this knowledge? In these days, we have to measure everything by utility — by how many pounds shillings, and pence it represents. What right has a person to ask that truth should be judged by the standard of utility or money? Suppose there is no utility, will it be less true? Utility is not the test of truth. Nevertheless, there is the highest utility in this. Happiness, we see is what everyone is seeking for, but the majority seek it in things which are evanescent and not real. No happiness was ever found in the senses. There never was a person who found happiness in the senses or in enjoyment of the senses. Happiness is only found in the Spirit. Therefore the highest utility for mankind is to find this happiness in the Spirit. The next point is that ignorance is the great mother of all misery, and the fundamental ignorance is to think that the Infinite weeps and cries, that He is finite. This is the basis of all ignorance that we, the immortal, the ever pure, the perfect Spirit, think that we are little minds, that we are little bodies; it is the mother of all selfishness. As soon as I think that I am a little body, I want to preserve it, to protect it, to keep it nice, at the expense of other bodies; then you and I become separate. As soon as this idea of separation comes, it opens the door to all mischief and leads to all misery. This is the utility that if a very small fractional part of human beings living today can put aside the idea of selfishness, narrowness, and littleness, this earth will become a paradise tomorrow; but with machines and improvements of material knowledge only, it will never be. These only increase misery, as oil poured on fire increases the flame all the more. Without the knowledge of the Spirit, all material knowledge is only adding fuel to fire, only giving into the hands of selfish man one more instrument to take what belongs to others, to live upon the life of others, instead of giving up his life for them.

Is it practical ? – is another question. Can it be practised in modern society? *Truth does not pay homage to any society, ancient or modern.* Society has to pay homage to Truth or die. *Societies should be moulded upon* truth, and truth has not to adjust itself to society. If such a noble truth as unselfishness cannot be practiced in society, it is better for man to give up society and go into the forest. That is the daring man. There are two sorts of courage. One is the courage of facing the cannon. And the other is the courage of spiritual conviction. An Emperor who invaded India was told by his teacher to go and see some of the sages there. After a long search for one, he found a very old man sitting on a block of stone. The Emperor talked with him a little and became very much impressed by his wisdom. He asked the sage to go to his country with him. "No," said the sage, "I am quite satisfied with my forest here." Said the Emperor, "I will give you money, position, wealth. I am the Emperor of the world." "No," replied the man, "I don't care for those things." The Emperor replied, "If you do not go, I will kill you." The man smiled serenely and said, "That is the most foolish thing you ever said, Emperor. You cannot kill me. Me the sun cannot dry, fire cannot burn, sword cannot kill, for I am the birthless, the deathless, the ever-living omnipotent, omnipresent Spirit." This is spiritual boldness, while the other is the courage of a lion or a tiger. In the Mutiny of 1857 there was a Swami, a very great soul, whom a Mohammedan mutineer stabbed severely. The Hindu mutineers caught and brought the man to the Swami, offering to kill him. But the Swami looked up calmly and said, "My brother, thou art He, thou art He!" and expired. This is another instance. What good is it to talk of the strength of your muscles, of the superiority of your Western institutions, if you cannot make Truth square with your society, if you cannot build up a society into which the highest Truth will fit? What is the good of this boastful talk about your grandeur and greatness, if you stand up and say, "This courage is not practical." Is nothing practical but pounds, shillings, and pence? If so, why boast of your society? *That society is the greatest, where the highest truths become* practical. *That is my opinion; and if society is; not fit for the highest* truths, make it so; and the sooner, the better. Stand up, men and women, in this spirit, dare to believe in the Truth, dare to practice the Truth! The world requires a few hundred bold men and women. Practise that boldness which dares know the Truth, which dares show the Truth in life, which does not quake before death, nay, welcomes death, makes a man know that he, is the Spirit, that, in the whole universe, nothing can kill him. Then you will be free. Then you will know yours real Soul. "This Atman is first to be heard, then thoughts about and then meditated upon."

There is a great tendency in modern times to talk too much of work and decry thought. Doing is very good, but that comes from thinking. Little manifestations of energy through the muscles are called work. But where there is no thought, there will be no work. Fill the brain, therefore, with high thoughts, highest ideals, place them day and night before you, and out of that will come great work. Talk not about impurity, but say that we are pure. We have hypnotised ourselves into this thought that we are little, that we are born, and that we are going to die, and into a constant state of fear.

There is a story about a lioness, who was big with young, going about in search of prey; and seeing a flock of sheep, she jumped upon them. She died in the effort; and a little baby lion was born, motherless. It was taken care of by the sheep and the sheep brought it up, and it grew up with them, ate grass, and bleated like the sheep. And although in time it became a big, full-grown lion. It thought it was a sheep. One day another lion came in search of prey and was astonished to find that in the midst of this flock of sheep was a lion, fleeing like the sheep at the approach of danger. He tried to get near the sheep-lion, to tell it that it was not a sheep but a lion; but the poor animal fled at his approach. However, he watched his opportunity and one day found the sheep-lion sleeping. He approached it and said, "You are a lion." "I am a sheep," cried the other lion and could not believe the contrary but bleated. The lion dragged him towards a lake and said, "Look here, here is my reflection and yours." Then came the comparison. It looked at the lion and then at its own reflection, and in a moment came the idea that it was a lion. The lion roared, the bleating was gone. You are lions, you are souls, pure, infinite, and perfect. The might of the universe is within you. "Why weepest thou, my friend? There is neither birth nor death for thee. Why weepest thou? There is no disease nor misery for thee, but thou art like the infinite sky; clouds of various colours come over it, play for a moment, then vanish. But the sky is ever the same eternal blue." Why do we see wickedness? There was a stump of a tree, and in the dark, a thief came that way and said, "That is a policeman." A young man waiting for his beloved saw it and thought that it was his sweetheart. A child who had been told ghost stories took it for a ghost and began to shriek. But all the time it was the stump of a tree. We see the world as we are. Suppose there is a baby in a room with a bag of gold on the table and a thief comes and steals the gold. Would the baby know it was stolen? That which we have inside, we see outside. The baby has no thief inside and sees no thief outside. So with all knowledge. Do not talk of the wickedness of the world and all its sins. Weep that you are bound to see wickedness yet. Weep that you are bound to see sin everywhere, and if you want to help the world, do not condemn it. Do not weaken it more. For what is sin and what is misery, and what are all these, but the results of weakness? The world is made weaker and weaker every day by such teachings. Men are taught from childhood that they are weak and sinners. Teach them that they are all glorious children of immortality, even those who are the weakest in manifestation. Let positive, strong, helpful thought enter into their brains from very childhood. Lay yourselves open to these thoughts, and not to weakening and paralysing ones. Say to your own minds, "I am He, I am He." Let it ring day and night in your minds like a song, and at the point of death declare "I am He." That is the Truth; the infinite strength of the world is yours. Drive out the superstition that has covered your minds. Let us be brave. Know the Truth and practice the Truth. The goal may be distant, but awake, arise, and stop not till the goal is reached.

❑

3

Maya and Illusion

(Delivered in London)

Almost all of you have heard of the word Mâyâ. Generally it is used, though incorrectly, to denote illusion, or delusion, or some such thing. But the theory of Maya forms one of the pillars upon which the Vedanta rests; it is, therefore, necessary that it should be properly understood. I ask a little patience of you, for there is a great danger of its being misunderstood. The oldest idea of Maya that we find in Vedic literature is the sense of delusion; but then the real theory had not been reached. We find such passages as, "Indra through his Maya assumed various forms." Here it is true the word Maya means something like magic, and we find various other passages, always taking the same meaning. The word Maya then dropped out of sight altogether. But in the meantime the idea was developing. Later, the question was raised: "Why can't we know this secret of the universe?" And the answer given was very significant: "Because we talk in vain, and because we are satisfied with the things of the senses, and because we are running after desires; therefore, we, as it were, cover the Reality with a mist." Here the word Maya is not used at all, but we get the idea that the cause of our ignorance is a kind of mist that has come between us and the Truth. Much later on, in one of the latest Upanishads, we find the word Maya reappearing, but this time, a transformation has taken place in it, and a mass of new meaning has attached itself to the word. Theories had been propounded and repeated, others had been taken up, until at last the idea of Maya became fixed. We read in the Shvetâshvatara Upanishad, "Know nature to be Maya and the Ruler of this Maya is the Lord Himself." Coming to our philosophers, we find that this word Maya has been manipulated in various fashions, until we come to the great Shankarâchârya. The theory of Maya was manipulated a little by the Buddhists too, but in the hands of the Buddhists it became very much like what is called Idealism, and that is the meaning that is now generally given to the word Maya. When the Hindu says the world is Maya, at once people get the idea that the world is an illusion. This interpretation has some basis, as coming through the Buddhistic philosophers, because there was one section of philosophers who did not believe in the external world at all. But the Maya of the Vedanta, in its last developed form, is neither Idealism nor Realism, nor is it a theory. It is a simple statement of facts – what we are and what we see around us.

As I have told you before, the minds of the people from whom the Vedas came were intent upon following principles, discovering principles. They had no time to work upon details or to wait for them; they wanted to go deep into the heart of things. Something beyond was calling them, as it were, and they could not wait. Scattered through the Upanishads, we find that the details of subjects which we now call modern sciences are often very erroneous, but, at the same time, their principles are correct. For instance, the idea of ether, which is one of the latest theories of modern science, is to be found in our ancient literature in forms much more developed than is the modern scientific theory of ether today, but it was in principle. When they tried to demonstrate the workings of that principle, they made many mistakes. The theory of the all-pervading life principle, of which all life in this universe is but a differing manifestation, was understood in Vedic times; it is found in the Brâhmanas. There is a long hymn in the Samhitâs in praise of Prâna of which all life is but a manifestation. By the by, it may interest some of you to know that there are theories in the Vedic philosophy about the origin of life on this earth very similar to those which have been advanced by some modern European scientists. You, of course, all know that there is a theory that life came from other planets. It is a settled doctrine with some Vedic philosophers that life comes in this way from the moon.

Coming to the principles, we find these Vedic thinkers very courageous and wonderfully bold in propounding large and generalised theories. Their solution of the mystery of the universe, from the external world, was as satisfactory as it could be. The detailed workings of modern science do not bring the question one step nearer to solution, because the principles have failed. If the theory of ether failed in ancient times to give a solution of the mystery of the universe, working out the details of that ether theory would not bring us much nearer to the truth. If the theory of all-pervading life failed as a theory of this universe, it would not mean anything more if worked out in detail, for the details do not change the principle of the universe. What I mean is that in their inquiry into the principle, the Hindu thinkers were as bold, and in some cases, much bolder than the moderns. They made some of the grandest generalizations that have yet been reached, and some still remain as theories, which modern science has yet to get even as theories. For instance, they not only arrived at the ether theory, but went beyond and classified mind also as a still more rarefied ether. Beyond that again, they found a still more rarefied ether. Yet that was no solution, it did not solve the problem. No amount of knowledge of the external world could solve the problem. "But", says the scientist, "we are just beginning to know a little: wait a few thousand years and we shall get the solution." "No," says the Vedantist, for he has proved beyond all doubt that the mind is limited, that it cannot go beyond certain limits – beyond time, space, and causation. As no man can jump out of his own self, so no man can go beyond the limits that have been put upon him by the laws of time and space. Every attempt to solve the laws of causation, time, and space would be futile, because the very attempt would have to be made by taking for granted the existence of these three. What does the statement of the existence of the world mean, then? "This world has no existence." What is meant by that? It means that it has no absolute existence. It exists only in relation to my mind, to your mind, and to the mind of everyone else. We see this world with the five senses but if we had another sense, we would see in it something more. If we had yet another sense, it would appear as something still different. It has, therefore, no real existence; it has no unchangeable, immovable, infinite existence. Nor can it be called non-existence, seeing that it exists, and we slave to work in and through it. It is a mixture of existence and non-existence.

Coming from abstractions to the common, everyday details of our lives, we find that our whole life is a contradiction, a mixture of existence and non-existence. There is this contradiction in knowledge. It seems that man can know everything, if he only wants to know; but before he has gone a few steps, he finds an adamantine wall which he cannot pass. All his work is in a circle, and he cannot go beyond that circle. The problems which are nearest and dearest to him are impelling him on and calling, day and night, for a solution, but he cannot solve them, because he cannot go beyond his intellect. And yet that desire is implanted strongly in him. Still we know that the only good is to be obtained by controlling and checking it. With every breath, every impulse of our heart asks us to be selfish. At the same time, there is some power beyond us which says that it is unselfishness alone which is good. Every child is a born optimist; he dreams golden dreams. In youth he becomes still more optimistic. It is hard for a young man to believe that there is such a thing as death, such a thing as defeat or degradation. Old age comes, and life is a mass of ruins. Dreams have vanished into the air, and the man becomes a pessimist. Thus we go from one extreme to another, buffeted by nature, without knowing where we are going. It reminds me of a celebrated song in the *Lalita Vistara*, the biography of Buddha. Buddha was born, says the book, as the saviour of mankind, but he forgot himself in the luxuries of his palace. Some angels came and sang a song to rouse him. And the burden of the whole song is that we are floating down the river of life which is continually changing with no stop and no rest. So are our lives, going on and on without knowing any rest. What are we to do? The man who has enough to eat and drink is an optimist, and he avoids all mention of misery, for it frightens him. Tell not to him of the sorrows and the sufferings of the world; go to him and tell that it is all good. "Yes, I am safe," says he. "Look at me! I have a nice house to live in. I do not fear cold and hunger; therefore do not bring these horrible pictures before me." But, on the other hand, there are others dying of cold and hunger. If you go and teach *them* that it is all good, they will not hear you. How can they wish others to be happy when they are miserable? Thus we are oscillating between optimism and pessimism.

Then, there is the tremendous fact of death. The whole world is going towards death; everything dies. All our progress, our vanities, our reforms, our luxuries, our wealth, our knowledge, have that one end — death. That is all that is certain. Cities come and go, empires rise and fall, planets break into pieces and crumble into dust, to be blown about by the atmospheres of other planets. Thus it has been going on from time without beginning. Death is the end of everything. Death is the end of life, of beauty, of wealth, of power, of virtue too. Saints die and sinners die, kings die and beggars die. They are all going to death, and yet this tremendous clinging on to life exists. Somehow, we do not know why, we cling to life; we cannot give it up. And this is Maya.

The mother is nursing a child with great care; all her soul, her life, is in that child. The child grows, becomes a man, and perchance becomes a blackguard and a brute, kicks her and beats her every day; and yet the mother clings to the child; and when her reason awakes, she covers it up with the idea of love. She little thinks that it is not love, that it is something which has got hold of her nerves, which she cannot shake off; however she may try, she cannot shake off the bondage she is in. And this is Maya.

We are all after the Golden Fleece. Every one of us thinks that this will be his. Every reasonable man sees that his chance is, perhaps, one in twenty millions, yet everyone struggles for it. And this is Maya.

Death is stalking day and night over this earth of ours, but at the same time we think we shall live eternally. A question was once asked of King Yudhishthira, "What is the most wonderful thing on this earth?" And the king replied, "Every day people are dying around us, and yet men think they will never die." And this is Maya.

These tremendous contradictions in our intellect, in our knowledge, yea, in all the facts of our life face us on all sides. A reformer arises and wants to remedy the evils that are existing in a certain nation; and before they have been remedied, a thousand other evils arise in another place. It is like an old house that is falling; you patch it up in one place and the ruin extends to another. In India, our reformers cry and preach against the evils of enforced widowhood. In the West, non-marriage is the great evil. Help the unmarried on one side; they are suffering. Help the widows on the other; they are suffering. It is like chronic rheumatism: you drive from the head, and it goes to the body; you drive it from there, and it goes to the feet. Reformers arise and preach that learning, wealth, and culture should not be in the hands of a select few; and they do their best to make them accessible to all. These may bring more happiness to some, but, perhaps, as culture comes, physical happiness lessens. The knowledge of happiness brings the knowledge of unhappiness. Which way then shall we go? The least amount of material prosperity that we enjoy is causing the same amount of misery elsewhere. This is the law. The young, perhaps, do not see it clearly, but those who have lived long enough and those who have struggled enough will understand it. And this is Maya. These things are going on, day and night, and to find a solution of this problem is impossible. Why should it be so? It is impossible to answer this, because the question cannot be logically formulated. There is neither *how* nor *why* in fact; we only know that it is and that we cannot help it. Even to grasp it, to draw an exact image of it in our own mind, is beyond our power. How can we solve it then?

Maya is a statement of the fact of this universe, of how it is going on. People generally get frightened when these things are told to them. But bold we must be. Hiding facts is not the way to find a remedy. As you all know, a hare hunted by dogs puts its head down and thinks itself safe; so, when we run into optimism; we do just like the hare, but that is no remedy. There are objections against this, but you may remark that they are generally from people who possess many of the good things of life. In this country (England) it is very difficult to become a pessimist. Everyone tells me how wonderfully the world is going on, how progressive; but what he himself is, is his own world. Old questions arise: Christianity must be the only true religion of the world because Christian nations are prosperous! But that assertion contradicts itself, because the prosperity of the Christian nation depends on the misfortune of non-Christian nations. There must be some to prey on. Suppose the whole world were to become Christian, then the Christian nations would become poor, because there would be no non-Christian nations for them to prey upon. Thus the argument kills itself. Animals are living upon plants, men upon animals and, worst of all, upon one another, the strong upon the weak. This is going on everywhere. And this is Maya. What solution do you find for this? We hear every day many explanations, and are told that in the long run all will be good. Taking it for granted that this is possible, why should there be this diabolical way of doing good? Why cannot good be done through good, instead of through these diabolical methods? The descendants of the human beings of today will be happy; but why must there be all this suffering now? There is no solution. This is Maya.

Again, we often hear that it is one of the features of evolution that it eliminates evil, and this evil being continually eliminated from the world, at last only good will remain. That is very nice to hear, and it panders to the vanity of those who have enough of this world's goods, who have not a hard struggle to face every clay and are not being crushed under the wheel of this so-called evolution. It is very good and comforting indeed to such fortunate ones. The common herd may surfer, but they do not care; let them die, they are of no consequence. Very good, yet this argument is fallacious from beginning to end. It takes for granted, in the first place, that manifested good and evil in this world are two absolute realities. In the second place, it make, at still worse assumption that the amount of good is an increasing quantity and the amount of evil is a decreasing quantity. So, if evil is being eliminated in this way by what they call evolution, there will come a time when all this evil will be eliminated and what remains will be all good. Very easy to say, but can it be proved that evil is a lessening quantity? Take, for instance, the man who lives in a forest, who does not know how to cultivate the mind, cannot read a book, has not heard of such a thing as writing. If he is severely wounded, he is soon all right again; while we die if we get a scratch. Machines are making things cheap, making for progress and evolution, but millions are crushed, that one may become rich; while one becomes rich, thousands at the same time become poorer and poorer, and whole masses of human beings are made slaves. That way it is going on. The animal man lives in the senses. If he does not get enough to eat, he is miserable; or if something happens to his body, he is miserable. In the senses both his misery and his happiness begin and end. As soon as this man progresses, as soon as his horizon of happiness increases, his horizon of unhappiness increases proportionately. The man in the forest does not know what it is to be jealous, to be in the law courts, to pay taxes, to be blamed by society, to be ruled over day and night by the most tremendous tyranny that human diabolism ever invented, which pries into the secrets of every human heart. He does not know how man becomes a thousand times more diabolical than any other animal, with all his vain knowledge and with all his pride. Thus it is that, as we emerge out of the senses, we develop higher powers of enjoyment, and at the same time we have to develop higher powers of suffering too. The nerves become finer and capable off more suffering. In every society, we often find that the ignorant, common man, when abused, does not feel much, but he feels a good thrashing. But the gentleman cannot bear a single word of abuse; he has become so finely nerved. Misery has increased with his susceptibility to happiness. This does not go much to prove the evolutionist's case. As we increase our power to be happy, we also increase our power to suffer, and sometimes I am inclined to think that if we increase our power to become happy in arithmetical progression, we shall increase, on the other hand, our power to become miserable in geometrical progression. We who are progressing know that the more we progress, the more avenues are opened to pain as well as to pleasure. And this is Maya.

Thus we find that Maya is not a theory for the explanation of the world; it is simply a statement of facts as they exist, that the very basis of our being is contradiction, that everywhere we have to move through this tremendous contradiction, that wherever there is good, there must also be evil, and wherever there is evil, there must be some good, wherever there is life, death must follow as its shadow, and everyone who smiles will have to weep, and vice versa. Nor can this state of things be remedied. We may verily imagine that there will be a place where there will be only good and no evil, where we shall only smile and never weep. This is impossible in the very nature of things; for the conditions will remain the same. Wherever there is the power of producing a smile in us, there lurks the power of producing tears. Wherever there is the power of producing happiness, there lurks somewhere the power of making us miserable.

Thus the Vedanta philosophy is neither optimistic nor pessimistic. It voices both these views and takes things as they are. It admits that this world is a mixture of good and evil, happiness and misery, and that to increase the one, one must of necessity increase the other. There will never be a perfectly good or bad world, because the very idea is a contradiction in terms. The great secret revealed by this analysis is that good and bad are not two cut-and-dried, separate existences. There is not one thing in this world of ours which you can label as good and good alone, and there is not one thing in the universe which you can label as bad and bad alone. The very same phenomenon which is appearing to be good now, may appear to be bad tomorrow. The same thing which is producing misery in one, may produce happiness in another. The fire that burns the child, may cook a good meal for a starving man. The same nerves that carry the sensations of misery carry also the sensations of happiness. The only way to stop evil, therefore, is to stop good also; there is no other way. To stop death, we shall have to stop life also. Life without death and happiness without misery are contradictions, and neither can be found alone, because each of them is but a different manifestation of the same thing. What I thought to be good yesterday, I do not think to be good now. When I look back upon my life and see what were my ideals at different times, I final this to be so. At one time my ideal was to drive a strong pair of horses; at another time I thought, if I could make a certain kind of sweetmeat, I should be perfectly happy; later I imagined that I should be entirely satisfied if I had a wife and children and plenty of money. Today I laugh at all these ideals as mere childish nonsense.

The Vedanta says, there must come a time when we shall look back and laugh at the ideals which make us afraid of giving up our individuality. Each one of us wants to keep this body for an indefinite time, thinking we shall be very happy, but there will come a time when we shall laugh at this idea. Now, if such be the truth, we are in a state of hopeless contradiction – neither existence nor non-existence, neither misery nor happiness, but a mixture of them. What, then, is the use of Vedanta and all other philosophies and religions? And, above all, what is the use of doing good work? This is a question that comes to the mind. If it is true that you cannot do good without doing evil, and whenever you try to create happiness there will always be misery, people will ask you, "What is the use of doing good?" The answer is in the first place, that we must work for lessening misery, for that is the only way to make ourselves happy. Every one of us finds it out sooner or later in our lives. The bright ones find it out a little earlier, and the dull ones a little later. The dull ones pay very dearly for the discovery and the bright ones less dearly. In the second place, we must do our part, because that is the only way of getting out of this life of contradiction. Both the forces of good and evil will keep the universe alive for us, until we awake from our dreams and give up this building of mud pies. That lesson we shall have to learn, and it will take a long, long time to learn it.

Attempts have been made in Germany to build a system of philosophy on the basis that the Infinite has become the finite. Such attempts are also made in England. And the analysis of the position of these philosophers is this, that the Infinite is trying to express itself in this universe, and that there will come a time when the Infinite will succeed in doing so. It is all very well, and we have used the words *Infinite* and *manifestation* and *expression*, and so on, but philosophers naturally ask for a logical fundamental basis for the statement that the finite can fully express the Infinite. The Absolute and the Infinite can become this universe only by limitation. Everything must be limited that comes through the senses, or through the mind, or through the intellect; and for the limited to be the unlimited is simply absurd and can never be. The Vedanta, on the other hand, says that it is true that the Absolute or the Infinite is trying to express itself in the finite, but there will come a time when it will find that it is impossible, and it will then have to beat a retreat, and this beating a retreat means renunciation which is the real beginning of religion. Nowadays it is very hard even to talk of renunciation. It was said of me in America that I was a man who came out of a land that had been dead and buried for five thousand years, and talked of renunciation. So says, perhaps, the English philosopher. Yet it is true that that is the only path to religion. Renounce and give up. What did Christ say? "He that loseth his life for my sake shall find it." Again and again did he preach renunciation as the only way to perfection. There comes a time when the mind awakes from this long and dreary dream — the child gives up its play and wants to go back to its mother. It finds the truth of the statement, "Desire is never satisfied by the enjoyment of desires, it only increases the more, as fire, when butter is poured upon it."

This is true of all sense-enjoyments, of all intellectual enjoyments, and of all the enjoyments of which the human mind is capable. They are nothing, they are within Maya, within this network beyond which we cannot go. We may run therein through infinite time and find no end, and whenever we struggle to get a little enjoyment, a mass of misery falls upon us. How awful is this! And when I think of it, I cannot but consider that this theory of Maya, this statement that it is all Maya, is the best and only explanation. What an amount of misery there is in this world; and if you travel among various nations you will find that one nation attempts to cure its evils by one means, and another by another. The very same evil has been taken up by various races, and attempts have been made in various ways to check it, yet no nation has succeeded. If it has been minimised at one point, a mass of evil has been crowded at another point. Thus it goes. The Hindus, to keep up a high standard of chastity in the race, have sanctioned child-marriage, which in the long run has degraded the race. At the same time, I cannot deny that this child-marriage makes the race more chaste. What would you have? If you want the nation to be more chaste, you weaken men and women physically by child-marriage. On the other hand, are you in England any better off? No, because chastity is the life of a nation. Do you not find in history that the first death-sign of a nation has been unchastity? When that has entered, the end of the race is in sight. Where shall we get a solution of these miseries then? If parents select husbands and wives for their children, then this evil is minimised. The daughters of India are more practical than sentimental. But very little of poetry remains in their lives. Again, if people select their own husbands and wives, that does not seem to bring much happiness. The Indian woman is generally very happy; there are not many cases of quarrelling between husband and wife. On the other hand in the United States, where the greatest liberty obtains, the number of unhappy homes and marriages is large. Unhappiness is here, there, and everywhere. What does it show? That, after all, not much happiness has been gained by all these ideals. We all struggle for happiness and as soon as we get a little happiness on one side, on the other side there comes unhappiness.

Shall we not work to do good then? Yes, with more zest than ever, but what this knowledge will do for us is to break down our fanaticism. The Englishman will no more be a fanatic and curse the Hindu. He will learn to respect the customs of different nations. There will be less of fanaticism and more of real work. Fanatics cannot work, they waste three-fourths of their energy. It is the level-headed, calm, practical man who works. So, the power to work will increase from this idea. Knowing that this is the state of things, there will be more patience. The sight of misery or of evil will not be able to throw us off our balance and make us run after shadows. Therefore, patience will come to us, knowing that the world will have to go on in its own way. If, for instance, all men have become good, the animals will have in the meantime evolved into men, and will have to pass through the same state, and so with the plants. But only one thing is certain; the mighty river is rushing towards the ocean, and all the drops that constitute the stream will in time be drawn into that boundless ocean. So, in this life, with all its miseries and sorrows, its joys and smiles and tears, one thing is certain, that all things are rushing towards their goal, and it: is only a question of time when you and I, and plants and animals, and every particles of life that exists must reach the Infinite Ocean of Perfection, must attain to Freedom, to God.

Let me repeat, once more, that the Vedantic position is neither pessimism nor optimism. It does not say that this world is all evil or all good. It says that our evil is of no less value than our good, and our good of no more value than our evil. They are bound together. This is the world, and knowing this, you work with patience. What for? Why should we work? If this is the state of things, what shall we do? Why not become agnostics? The modern agnostics also know there is no solution of this problem, no getting out of this evil of Maya, as we say in our language; therefore they tell us to be satisfied and enjoy life. Here, again, is a mistake, a tremendous mistake, a most illogical mistake. And it is this. What do you mean by life? Do you mean only the life of the senses? In this, every one of us differs only slightly from the brutes. I am sure that no one is present here whose life is only in the senses. Then, this present life means something more than that. Our feelings, thoughts, and aspirations are all part and parcel of our life; and is not the struggle towards the area, ideal, towards perfection, one of the most important components of what we call life? According to the agnostics, we must enjoy life as it is. But this life means, above all, this search after the ideal; the essence of life is going towards perfection. We must have that, and, therefore, we cannot be agnostics or take the world as it appears. The agnostic position takes this life, minus the ideal component, to be all that exists. And this, the agnostic claims, cannot be reached, therefore he must give up the search. This is what is called Maya — this nature, this universe.

All religions are more or less attempts to get beyond nature — the crudest or the most developed, expressed through mythology or symbology, stories of gods, angels or demons, or through stories of saints or seers, great men or prophets, or through the abstractions of philosophy — all have that one object, all are trying to get beyond these limitations. In one word, they are all struggling towards freedom. Man feels, consciously or unconsciously, that he is bound; he is not what he wants to be. It was taught to him at the very moment he began to look around. That very instant he learnt that he was bound, and be also found that there was something in him which wanted to fly beyond, where the body could not follow, but which was as yet chained down by this limitation. Even in the lowest of religious ideas, where departed ancestors and other spirits — mostly violent and cruel, lurking about the houses of their friends, fond of bloodshed and strong drink — are worshipped, even there we find that one common factor, that of freedom. The man who wants to worship the gods sees in them, above all things, greater freedom than in himself. If a door is closed, he thinks the gods can get through it, and that walls have no limitations for them. This idea of freedom increases until it comes to the ideal of a Personal God, of which the central concept is that He is a Being beyond the limitation of nature, of Maya. I see before me, as it were, that in some of those forest retreats this question is being, discussed by those ancient sages of India; and in one of them, where even the oldest and the holiest fail to reach the solutions a young man stands up in the midst of them, and declares, "Hear, ye children of immortality, hear, who live in the highest places, I have found the way. By knowing Him who is beyond darkness we can go beyond death."

This Maya is everywhere. It is terrible. Yet we have to work through it. The man who says that he will work when the world has become all good and then he will enjoy bliss is as likely to succeed as the man who sits beside the Ganga and says, "I will ford the river when all the water has run into the ocean." The way is not with Maya, but against it. This is another fact to learn. We are not born as helpers of nature, but competitors with nature. We are its bond-masters, but we bind ourselves down. Why is this house here? Nature did not build it. Nature says, go and live in the forest. Man says, I will build a house and fight with nature, and he does so. The whole history of humanity is a continuous fight against the so-called laws of nature, and man gains in the end. Coming to the internal world, there too the same fight is going on, this fight between the animal man and the spiritual man, between light and darkness; and here too man becomes victorious. He, as it were, cuts his way out of nature to freedom.

We see, then, that beyond this Maya the Vedantic philosophers find something which is not bound by Maya; and if we can get there, we shall not be bound by Maya. This idea is in some form or other the common property of all religions. But, with the Vedanta, it is only the beginning of religion and not the end. The idea of a Personal God, the Ruler and Creator of this universe, as He has been styled, the Ruler of Maya, or nature, is not the end of these Vedantic ideas; it is only the beginning. The idea grows and grows until the Vedantist finds that He who, he thought, was standing outside, is he himself and is in reality within. He is the one who is free, but who through limitation thought he was bound.

❑

4

Maya and the Evolution of the Conception of God

(Delivered in London, 20th October 1896)

We have seen how the idea of Mâyâ, which forms, as it were, one of the basic doctrines of the Advaita Vedanta, is, in its germs, found even in the Samhitâs, and that in reality all the ideas which are developed in the Upanishads are to be found already in the Samhitas in some form or other. Most of you are by this time familiar with the idea of Maya, and know that it is sometimes erroneously explained as illusion, so that when the universe is said to be Maya, that also has to be explained as being illusion. The translation of the word is neither happy nor correct. Maya is not a theory; it is simply a statement of facts about the universe as it exists, and to understand Maya we must go back to the Samhitas and begin with the conception in the germ.

We have seen how the idea of the Devas came. At the same time we know that these Devas were at first only powerful beings, nothing more. Most of you are horrified when reading the old scriptures, whether of the Greeks, the Hebrews, the Persians, or others, to find that the ancient gods sometimes did things which, to us, are very repugnant. But when we read these books, we entirely forget that we are persons of the nineteenth century, and these gods were beings existing thousands of years ago. We also forget that the people who worshipped these gods found nothing incongruous in their characters, found nothing to frighten them, because they were very much like themselves. I may also remark that that is the one great lesson we have to learn throughout our lives. In judging others we always judge them by our own ideals. That is not as it should be. Everyone must be judged according to his own ideal, and not by that of anyone else. In our dealings with our fellow-beings we constantly labour under this mistake, and I am of opinion that the vast majority of our quarrels with one another arise simply from this one cause that we are always trying to judge others' gods by our own, others' ideals by our ideals, and others' motives by our motives. Under certain circumstances I might do a certain thing, and when I see another person taking the same course I think he has also the same motive actuating him, little dreaming that although the effect may be the same, yet many other causes may produce the same thing. He may have performed the action with quite a different motive from that which impelled me to do it. So in judging of those ancient religions we must not take the standpoint to which we incline, but must put ourselves into the position of thought and life of those early times.

The idea of the cruel and ruthless Jehovah in the Old Testament has frightened many — but why? What right have they to assume that the Jehovah of the ancient Jews must represent the conventional idea of the God of the present day? And at the same time, we must not forget that there will come men after us who will laugh at our ideas of religion and God in the same way that we laugh at those of the ancients. Yet, through all these various conceptions runs the golden thread of unity, and it is the purpose of the Vedanta to discover this thread. "I am the thread that runs through all these various ideas, each one of which is; like a pearl," says the Lord Krishna; and it is the duty of Vedanta to establish this connecting thread, how ever incongruous or disgusting may seem these ideas when judged according to the conceptions of today. These ideas, in the setting of past times, were harmonious and not more hideous than our present ideas. It is only when we try to take them out of their settings and apply to our own present circumstances that the hideousness becomes obvious. For the old surroundings are dead and gone. Just as the ancient Jew has developed into the keen, modern, sharp Jew, and the ancient Aryan into the intellectual Hindu similarly Jehovah has grown, and Devas have grown.

The great mistake is in recognising the evolution of the worshippers, while we do not acknowledge the evolution of the Worshipped. He is not credited with the advance that his devotees have made. That is to say, you and I, representing ideas, have grown; these gods also, as representing ideas, have grown. This may seem somewhat curious to you — that God can grow. He cannot. He is unchangeable. In the same sense the real man never grows. But man's ideas of God are constantly changing and expanding. We shall see later on how the real man behind each one of these human manifestations is immovable, unchangeable, pure, and always perfect; and in the same way the idea that we form of God is a mere manifestation, our own creation. Behind that is the real God who never changes, the ever pure, the immutable. But the manifestation is always changing revealing the reality behind more and more. When it reveals more of the fact behind, it is called progression, when it hides more of the fact behind, it is called retrogression. Thus, as we grow, so the gods grow. From the ordinary point of view, just as we reveal ourselves as we evolve, so the gods reveal themselves.

We shall now be in a position to understand the theory of Maya. In all the regions of the world the one question they propose to discuss is this: Why is there disharmony in the universe? Why is there this evil in the universe? We do not find this question in the very inception of primitive religious ideas, because the world did not appear incongruous to the primitive man. Circumstances were not inharmonious for him; there was no dash of opinions; to him there was no antagonism of good and evil. There was merely a feeling in his own heart of something which said yea, and something which said nay. The primitive man was a man of impulse. He did what occurred to him, and tried to bring out through his muscles whatever thought came into his mind, and he never stopped to judge, and seldom tried to check his impulses. So with the gods, they were also creatures of impulse. Indra comes and shatters the forces of the demons. Jehovah is pleased with one person and displeased with another, for what reason no one knows or asks. The habit of inquiry had not then arisen, and whatever he did was regarded as right. There was no idea of good or evil. The

Devas did many wicked things in our sense of the word; again and again Indra and other gods committed very wicked deeds, but to the worshippers of Indra the ideas of wickedness and evil did not occur, so they did not question them.

With the advance of ethical ideas came the fight. There arose a certain sense in man, called in different languages and nations by different names. Call it the voice of God, or the result of past education, or whatever else you like, but the effect was this that it had a checking power upon the natural impulses of man. There is one impulse in our minds which says, do. Behind it rises another voice which says, do not. There is one set of ideas in our mind which is always struggling to get outside through the channels of the senses, and behind that, although it may be thin and weak, there is an infinitely small voice which says, do not go outside. The two beautiful Sanskrit words for these phenomena are Pravritti and Nivritti, "circling forward" and "circling inward". It is the circling forward which usually governs our actions. Religion begins with this circling inward. Religion begins with this "do not". Spirituality begins with this "do not". When the "do not" is not there, religion has not begun. And this "do not" came, causing men's ideas to grow, despite the fighting gods which they had worshipped.

A little love awoke in the hearts of mankind. It was very small indeed, and even now it is not much greater. It was at first confined to a tribe embracing perhaps members of the same tribe; these gods loved their tribes and each god was a tribal god, the protector of that tribe. And sometimes the members of a tribe would think of themselves as the descendants of their god, just as the clans in different nations think that they are the common descendants of the man who was the founder of the clan. There were in ancient times, and are even now, some people who claim to be descendants not only of these tribal gods, but also of the Sun and the Moon. You read in the ancient Sanskrit books of the great heroic emperors of the solar and the lunar dynasties. They were first worshippers of the Sun and the Moon, and gradually came to think of themselves as descendants of the god of the Sun of the Moon, and so forth. So when these tribal ideas began to grow there came a little love, some slight idea of duty towards each other, a little social organisation. Then, naturally, the idea came: How can we live together without bearing and forbearing? How can one man live with another without having some time or other to check his impulses, to restrain himself, to forbear from doing things which his mind would prompt him to do? It is impossible. Thus comes the idea of restraint. The whole social fabric is based upon that idea of restraint, and we all know that the man or woman who has not learnt the great lesson of bearing and forbearing leads a most miserable life.

Now, when these ideas of religion came, a glimpse of something higher, more ethical, dawned upon the intellect of mankind. The old gods were found to be incongruous – these boisterous, fighting, drinking, beef-eating gods of the ancients – whose delight was in the smell of burning flesh and libations of strong liquor. Sometimes Indra drank so much that he fell upon the ground and talked unintelligibly. These gods could no longer be tolerated. The notion had arisen of inquiring into motives, and the gods had to come in for their share of inquiry. Reason for such-and-such actions was demanded and the reason was wanting. Therefore man gave up these gods, or rather they developed higher ideas concerning them. They took a survey, as it were, of all the actions and qualities of the gods and discarded those which they could not harmonise, and kept those which they could understand, and combined them, labelling them with one name, Deva-deva, the God of gods. The god to be worshipped was no more a simple symbol of power; something more was required than that. He was an ethical god; he loved mankind, and did good to mankind. But the idea of god still remained. They increased his ethical significance, and increased also his power. He became the most ethical being in the universe, as well as almost almighty.

But all this patchwork would not do. As the explanation assumed greater proportions, the difficulty which it sought to solve did the same. If the qualities of the god increased in arithmetical progression, the difficulty and doubt increased in geometrical progression. The difficulty of Jehovah was very little beside the difficulty of the God of the universe, and this question remains to the present day. Why under the reign of an almighty and all-loving God of the universe should diabolical things be allowed to remain? Why so much more misery than happiness, and so much more wickedness than good? We may shut our eyes to all these things, but the fact still remains that this world is a hideous world. At best, it is the hell of Tantalus. Here we are with strong impulses and stronger cravings for sense-enjoyments, but cannot satisfy them. There rises a wave which impels us forward in spite of our own will, and as soon as we move one step, comes a blow. We are all doomed to live here like Tantalus. Ideals come into our head far beyond the limit of our sense-ideals, but when we seek to express them, we cannot do so. On the other hand, we are crushed by the surging mass around us. Yet if I give up all ideality and merely struggle through this world, my existence is that of a brute, and I degenerate and degrade myself. Neither way is happiness. Unhappiness is the fate of those who are content to live in this world, born as they are. A thousand times greater misery is the fate of those who dare to stand forth for truth and for higher things and who dare to ask for something higher than mere brute existence here. These are facts; but there is no explanation — there cannot be any explanation. But the Vedanta shows the way out. You must bear in mind that I have to tell you facts that will frighten you sometimes, but if you remember what I say, think of it, and digest it, it will be yours, it will raise you higher, and make you capable of understanding and living in truth.

Now, it is a statement of fact that this world is a Tantalus's hell, that we do not know anything about this universe, yet at the same time we cannot say that we do not know. I cannot say that this chain exists, when I think that I do not know it. It may be an entire delusion of my brain. I may be dreaming all the time. I am dreaming that I am talking to you, and that you are listening to me. No one can prove that it is not a dream. My brain itself may be a dream, and as to that no one has ever seen his own brain. We all take it for granted. So it is with everything. My own body I take for granted. At the same time I cannot say, I do not know. This standing between knowledge and ignorance, this mystic twilight, the mingling of truth and falsehood — and where they meet — no one knows. We are walking in the midst of a dream. Half sleeping, half waking, passing all our lives in a haze; this is the fate of everyone of us. This is the fate of all sense-knowledge. This is the fate of all philosophy, of all boasted science, of all boasted human knowledge. This is the universe.

What you call matter, or spirit, or mind, or anything else you may like to call them, the fact remains the same: we cannot say that they are, we cannot say that they are not. We cannot say they are one, we cannot say they are many. This eternal play of light and darkness – indiscriminate, indistinguishable, inseparable – is always there. A fact, yet at the same time not a fact; awake and at the same time asleep. This is a statement of facts, and this is what is called Maya. We are born in this Maya, we live in it, we think in it, we dream in it. We are philosophers in it, we are spiritual men in it, nay, we are devils in this Maya, and we are gods in this Maya. Stretch your ideas as far as you can make them higher and higher, call them infinite or by any other name you please, even these ideas are within this Maya. It cannot be otherwise, and the whole of human knowledge is a generalization of this Maya trying to know it as it appears to be. This is the work of Nâma-Rupa – name and form. Everything that has form, everything that calls up an idea in your mind, is within Maya; for everything that is bound by the laws of time, space, and causation is within Maya.

Let us go back a little to those early ideas of God and see what became of them. We perceive at once that the idea of some Being who is eternally loving us – eternally unselfish and almighty, ruling this universe – could not satisfy. "Where is the just, merciful God?" asked the philosopher. Does He not see millions and millions of His children perish, in the form of men and animals; for who can live one moment here without killing others? Can you draw a breath without destroying thousands of lives? You live, because, millions die. Every moment of your life, every breath that you breathe, is death to thousands; every movement that you make is death to millions. Every morsel that you eat is death to millions. Why should they die? There is an old sophism that they are very low existences. Supposing they are – which is questionable, for who knows whether the ant is greater than the man, or the man than the ant — who can prove one way or the other? Apart from that question, even taking it for granted that these are very low beings, still why should they die? If they are low, they have more reason to live. Why not? Because they live more in the senses, they feel pleasure and pain a thousandfold more than you or I can do. Which of us eats a dinner with the same gusto as a dog or wolf? None, because our energies are not in the senses; they are in the intellect, in the spirit. But in animals, their whole soul is in the senses, and they become mad and enjoy things which we human beings never dream of, and the pain is commensurate with the pleasure. Pleasure and pain are meted out in equal measure. If the pleasure felt by animals is so much keener than that felt by man, it follows that the animals' sense of pain is as keen, if not keener than man's. So the fact is, the pain and misery men feel in dying is intensified a thousandfold in animals, and yet we kill them without troubling ourselves about their misery. This is Maya. And if we suppose there is a Personal God like a human being, who made everything, these so-called explanations and theories which try to prove that out of evil comes good are not sufficient. Let twenty thousand good things come, but why should they come from evil? On that principle, I might cut the throats of others because I want the full pleasure of my five senses. That is no reason. Why should good come through evil? The question remains to be answered, and it cannot be answered. The philosophy of India was compelled to admit this.

The Vedanta was (and is) the boldest system of religion. It stopped nowhere, and it had one advantage. There was no body of priests who sought to suppress every man who tried to tell the truth. There was always absolute religious freedom. In India the bondage of superstition is a social one; here in the West society is very free. Social matters in India are very strict, but religious opinion is free. In England a man may dress any way he likes, or eat what he lilies — no one objects; but if he misses attending church, then Mrs. Grundy is down on him. He has to conform first to what society says on religion, and then he may think of the truth. In India, on the other hand, if a man dines with one who does not belong to his own caste, down comes society with all its terrible powers and crushes him then and there. If he wants to dress a little differently from the way in which his ancestor dressed ages ago, he is done for. I have heard of a man who was cast out by society because he went several miles to see the first railway train. Well, we shall presume that was not true! But in religion, we find atheists, materialists, and Buddhists, creeds, opinions, and speculations of every phase and variety, some of a most startling character, living side by side. Preachers of all sects go about reaching and getting adherents, and at the very gates of the temples of gods, the Brâhmins – to their credit be it said – allow even the materialists to stand and give forth their opinions.

Buddha died at a ripe old age. I remember a friend of mine, a great American scientist, who was fond of reading his life. He did not like the death of Buddha, because he was not crucified. What a false idea! For a man to be great he must be murdered! Such ideas never prevailed in India. This great Buddha travelled all over India, denouncing her gods and even the God of the universe, and yet he lived to a good old age. For eighty years he lived, and had converted half the country.

Then, there were the Chârvâkas, who preached horrible things, the most rank, undisguised materialism, such as in the nineteenth century they dare not openly preach. These Charvakas were allowed to preach from temple to temple, and city to city, that religion was all nonsense, that it was priestcraft, that the Vedas were the words and writings of fools, rogues, and demons, and that there was neither God nor an eternal soul. If there was a soul, why did it not come back after death drawn by the love of wife and child. Their idea was that if there was a soul it must still love after death, and want good things to eat and nice dress. Yet no one hurt these Charvakas.

Thus India has always had this magnificent idea of religious freedom, and you must remember that freedom is the first condition of growth. What you do not make free, will never grow. The idea that you can make others grow and help their growth, that you can direct and guide them, always retaining for yourself the freedom of the teacher, is nonsense, a dangerous lie which has retarded the growth of millions and millions of human beings in this world. Let men have the light of liberty. That is the only condition of growth.

We, in India, allowed liberty in spiritual matters, and we have a tremendous spiritual power in religious thought even today. You grant the same liberty in social matters, and so have a splendid social organisation. We have not given any freedom to the expansion of social matters, and ours is a cramped society. You have never given any freedom in religious matters but with fire and sword have enforced your beliefs, and the result is that religion is a stunted, degenerated growth in the European mind. In India, we have to take off the shackles from society; in Europe, the chains must be taken from the feet of spiritual progress. Then will come a wonderful growth and development of man. If we discover that there is one unity running through all these developments, spiritual, moral, and social, we shall find that religion, in the fullest sense of the word, must come into society, and into our everyday life. In the light of Vedanta you will Understand that all sciences are but manifestations of religion, and so is everything that exists in this world.

We see, then, that through freedom the sciences were built; and in them we have two sets of opinions, the one the materialistic and denouncing, and the other the positive and constructive. It is a most curious fact that in every society you find them. Supposing there is an evil in society, you will find immediately one group rise up and denounce it in vindictive fashion, which sometimes degenerates into fanaticism. There are fanatics in every society, and women frequently join in these outcries, because of their impulsive nature. Every fanatic who gets up and denounces something can secure a following. It is very easy to break down; a maniac can break anything he likes, but it would be hard for him to build up anything. These fanatics may do some good, according to their light, but much morn harm. Because social institutions are not made in a day, and to change them means removing the cause. Suppose there is an evil; denouncing it will not remove it, but you must go to work at the root. First find out the cause, then remove it, and the effect will be removed also. Mere outcry not produce any effect, unless indeed it produces misfortune.

There are others who had sympathy in their hearts and who understood the idea that we must go deep into the cause, these were the great saints. One fact you must remember, that all the great teachers of the world have declared that they came not to destroy but to fulfil. Many times his has not been understood, and their forbearance has been thought to be an unworthy compromise with existing popular opinions. Even now, you occasionally hear that these prophets and great teachers were rather cowardly, and dared not say and do what they thought was right; but that was not so. Fanatics little understand the infinite power of love in the hearts of these great sages who looked upon the inhabitants of this world as their children. They were the real fathers, the real gods, filled with infinite sympathy and patience for everyone; they were ready to bear and forbear. They knew how human society should grow, and patiently slowly, surely, went on applying their remedies, not by denouncing and frightening people, but by gently and kindly leading them upwards step by step. Such were the writers of the Upanishads. They knew full well how the old ideas of God were not reconcilable with the advanced ethical ideas of the time; they knew full well that what the atheists were preaching contained a good deal of truth, nay, great nuggets of truth; but at the same time, they understood that those who wished to sever the thread that bound the beads, who wanted to build a new society in the air, would entirely fail.

We never build anew, we simply change places; we cannot have anything new, we only change the position of things. The seed grows into the tree, patiently and gently; we must direct our energies towards the truth and fulfil the truth that exists, not try to make new truths. Thus, instead of denouncing these old ideas of God as unfit for modern times, the ancient sages began to seek out the reality that was in them. The result was the Vedanta philosophy, and out of the old deities, out of the monotheistic God, the Ruler of the universe, they found yet higher and higher ideas in what is called the Impersonal Absolute; they found oneness throughout the universe.

He who sees in this world of manifoldness that One running through all, in this world of death he who finds that One Infinite Life, and in this world of insentience and ignorance he who finds that One Light and Knowledge, unto him belongs eternal peace. Unto none else, unto none else.

❑

5

Maya and Freedom

(Delivered in London, 22nd October 1896)

"Trailing clouds of glory we come," says the poet. Not all of us come as trailing clouds of glory however; some of us come as trailing black fogs; there can be no question about that. But every one of us comes into this world to fight, as on a battlefield. We come here weeping to fight our way, as well as we can, and to make a path for ourselves through this infinite ocean of life; forward we go, having long ages behind us and an immense expanse beyond. So on we go, till death comes and takes us off the field – victorious or defeated, we do not know. And this is Mâyâ.

Hope is dominant in the heart of childhood. The whole world is a golden vision to the opening eyes of the child; he thinks his will is supreme. As he moves onward, at every step nature stands as an adamantine wall, barring his future progress. He may hurl himself against it again and again, striving to break through. The further he goes, the further recedes the ideal, till death comes, and there is release, perhaps. And this is Maya.

A man of science rises, he is thirsting after knowledge. No sacrifice is too great, no struggle too hopeless for him. He moves onward discovering secret after secret of nature, searching out the secrets from her innermost heart, and what for? What is it all for? Why should we give him glory? Why should he acquire fame? Does not nature do infinitely more than any human being can do? – and nature is dull, insentient. Why should it be glory to imitate the dull, the insentient? Nature can hurl a thunderbolt of any magnitude to any distance. If a man can do one small part as much, we praise him and laud him to the skies. Why? Why should we praise him for imitating nature, imitating death, imitating dullness imitating insentience? The force of gravitation can pull to pieces the biggest mass that ever existed; yet it is insentient. What glory is there in imitating the insentient? Yet we are all struggling after that. And this is maya.

The senses drag the human soul out. Man is seeking for pleasure and for happiness where it can never be found. For countless ages we are all taught that this is futile and vain, there is no happiness here. But we cannot learn; it is impossible for us to do so, except through our own experiences. We try them, and a blow comes. Do we learn then? Not even then. Like moths hurling themselves against the flame, we are hurling ourselves again and again into sense-pleasures, hoping to find satisfaction there. We return again and again with freshened energy; thus we go on, till crippled and cheated we die. And this is Maya.

So with our intellect. In our desire to solve the mysteries of the universe, we cannot stop our questioning, we feel we must know and cannot believe that no knowledge is to be gained. A few steps, and there arises the wall of beginningless and endless time which we cannot surmount. A few steps, and there appears a wall of boundless space which cannot be surmounted, and the whole is irrevocably bound in by the walls of cause and effect. We cannot go beyond them. Yet we struggle, and still have to struggle. And this is Maya.

With every breath, with every pulsation of the heart with every one of our movements, we think we are free, and the very same moment we are shown that we are not. Bound slaves, nature's bond-slaves, in body, in mind, in all our thoughts, in all our feelings. And this is Maya.

There was never a mother who did not think her child was a born genius, the most extraordinary child that was ever born; she dotes upon her child. Her whole soul is in the child. The child grows up, perhaps becomes a drunkard, a brute, ill-treats the mother, and the more he ill-treats her, the more her love increases. The world lauds it as the unselfish love of the mother, little dreaming that the mother is a born slave, she cannot help it. She would a thousand times rather throw off the burden, but she cannot. So she covers it with a mass of flowers, which she calls wonderful love. And this is Maya.

We are all like this in the world. A legend tells how once Nârada said to Krishna, "Lord, show me Maya." A few days passed away, and Krishna asked Narada to make a trip with him towards a desert, and after walking for several miles, Krishna said, "Narada, I am thirsty; can you fetch some water for me?" "I will go at once, sir, and get you water." So Narada went. At a little distance there was a village; he entered the village in search of water and knocked at a door, which was opened by a most beautiful young girl. At the sight of her he immediately forgot that his Master was waiting for water, perhaps dying for the want of it. He forgot everything and began to talk with the girl. All that day he did not return to his Master. The next day, he was again at the house, talking to the girl. That talk ripened into love; he asked the father for the daughter, and they were married and lived there and had children. Thus twelve years passed. His father-in-law died, he inherited his property. He lived, as he seemed to think, a very happy life with his wife and children, his fields and his cattle and so forth. Then came a flood. One night the river rose until it overflowed its banks and flooded the whole village. Houses fell, men and animals were swept away and drowned, and everything was floating in the rush of the stream. Narada had to escape. With one hand be held his wife, and with the other two of his children; another child was on his shoulders, and he was trying to ford this tremendous flood. After a few steps he found the current was too strong, and the child on his shoulders fell and was borne away. A cry of despair came from Narada. In trying to save that child, he lost his grasp upon one of the others, and it also was lost. At last his wife, whom he clasped with all his might, was torn away by the current, and he was thrown on the bank, weeping and wailing in bitter lamentation. Behind him there came a gentle voice, "My child, where is the water? You went to fetch a pitcher of water, and I am waiting for you; you have been gone for quite half an hour." "Half an hour! " Narada exclaimed. Twelve whole years had passed through his mind, and all these scenes had happened in half an hour! And this is Maya.

In one form or another, we are all in it. It is a most difficult and intricate state of things to understand. It has been preached in every country, taught everywhere, but only believed in by a few, because until we get the experiences ourselves we cannot believe in it. What does it show? Something very terrible. For it is all futile. Time, the avenger of everything, comes, and nothing is left. He swallows up the saint and the sinner, the king and the peasant, the beautiful and the ugly; he leaves nothing. Everything is rushing towards that one goal destruction. Our knowledge, our arts, our sciences, everything is rushing towards it. None can stem the tide, none can hold it back for a minute. We may try to forget it, in the same way that persons in a plague-striker city try to create oblivion by drinking, dancing, and other vain attempts, and so becoming paralysed. So we are trying to forget, trying to create oblivion by all sorts of sense-pleasures. And this is Maya.

Two ways have been proposed. One method, which everyone knows, is very common, and that is: "It may be very true, but do not think of it. 'Make hay while the sun shines,' as the proverb says. It is all true, it is a fact, but do not mind it. Seize the few pleasures you can, do what little you can, do not look at tile dark side of the picture, but always towards the hopeful, the positive side." There is some truth in this, but there is also a danger. The truth is that it is a good motive power. Hope and a positive ideal are very good motive powers for our lives, but there is a certain danger in them. The danger lies in our giving up the struggle in despair. Such is the case with those who preach, "Take the world as it is, sit down as calmly and comfortably as you can and be contented with all these miseries. When you receive blows, say they are not blows but flowers; and when you are driven about like slaves, say that you are free. Day and night tell lies to others and to your own souls, because that is the only way to live happily." This is what is called practical wisdom, and never was it more prevalent in the world than in this nineteenth century; because never were harder blows hit than at the present time, never was competition keener, never were men so cruel to their fellow-men as now; and, therefore, must this consolation be offered. It is put forward in the strongest way at the present time; but it fails, as it always must fail. We cannot hide a carrion with roses; it is impossible. It would not avail long; for soon the roses would fade, and the carrion would be worse than ever before. So with our lives. We may try to cover our old and festering sores with cloth of gold, but there comes a day when the cloth of gold is removed, and the sore in all its ugliness is revealed.

Is there no hope then? True it is that we are all slaves of Maya, born in Maya, and live in Maya. Is there then no way out, no hope? That we are all miserable, that this world is really a prison, that even our so-called trailing beauty is but a prison-house, and that even our intellects and minds are prison-houses, have been known for ages upon ages. There has never been a man, there has never been a human soul, who has not felt this sometime or other, however he may talk. And the old people feel it most, because in them is the accumulated experience of a whole life, because they cannot be easily cheated by the lies of nature. Is there no way out? We find that with all this, with this terrible fact before us, in the midst of sorrow and suffering, even in this world where life and death are synonymous, even here, there is a still small voice that is ringing through all ages, through every country, and in every heart: "This My Maya is divine, made up of qualities, and very difficult to cross. Yet those that come unto Me, cross the river of life." "Come unto Me all ye that labour and are heavy laden and I will give you rest." This is the voice that is leading us forward. Man has heard it, and is hearing it all through the ages. This voice comes to men when everything seems to be lost and hope has fled, when man's dependence on his own strength has been crushed down and everything seems to melt away between his fingers, and life is a hopeless ruin. Then he hears it. This is called religion.

On the one side, therefore, is the bold assertion that this is all nonsense, that this is Maya, but along with it there is the most hopeful assertion that beyond Maya, there is a way out. On the other hand, practical men tell us, "Don't bother your heads about such nonsense as religion and metaphysics. Live here; this is a very bad world indeed, but make the best of it." Which put in plain language means, live a hypocritical, lying life, a life of continuous fraud, covering all sores in the best way you can. Go on putting patch after patch, until everything is lost, and you are a mass of patchwork. This is what is called practical life. Those that are satisfied with this patchwork will never come to religion. Religion begins with a tremendous dissatisfaction with the present state of things, with our lives, and a hatred, an intense hatred, for this patching up of life, an unbounded disgust for fraud and lies. He alone can be religious who dares say, as the mighty Buddha once said under the Bo-tree, when this idea of practicality appeared before him and he saw that it was nonsense, and yet could not find a way out. When the temptation came to him to give up his search after truth, to go back to the world and live the old life of fraud, calling things by wrong names, telling lies to oneself and to everybody, he, the giant, conquered it and said, "Death is better than a vegetating ignorant life; it is better to die on the battle-field than to live a life of defeat." This is the basis of religion. When a man takes this stand, he is on the way to find the truth, he is on the way to God. That determination must be the first impulse towards becoming religious. I will hew out a way for myself. I will know the truth or give up my life in the attempt. For on this side it is nothing, it is gone, it is vanishing every day. The beautiful, hopeful, young person of today is the veteran of tomorrow. Hopes and joys and pleasures will die like blossoms with tomorrow's frost. That is one side; on the other, there are the great charms of conquest, victories over all the ills of life, victory over life itself, the conquest of the universe. On that side men can stand. Those who dare, therefore, to struggle for victory, for truth, for religion, are in the right way; and that is what the Vedas preach: Be not in despair, the way is very difficult, like walking on the edge of a razor; yet despair not, arise, awake, and find the ideal, the goal.

Now all these various manifestations of religion, in whatever shape and form they have come to mankind, have this one common central basis. It is the preaching of freedom, the way out of this world. They never came to reconcile the world and religion, but to cut the Gordian knot, to establish religion in its own ideal, and not to compromise with the world. That is what every religion preaches, and the duty of the Vedanta is to harmonise all these aspirations, to make manifest the common ground between all the religions of the world, the highest as well as the lowest. What we call the most arrant superstition and the highest philosophy really have a common aim in that they both try to show the way out of the same difficulty, and in most cases this way is through the help of someone who is not himself bound by the laws of nature in one word, someone who is free. In spite of all the difficulties and differences of opinion about the nature of the one free agent, whether he is a Personal God, or a sentient being like man, whether masculine, feminine, or neuter – and the discussions have been endless – the fundamental idea is the same. In spite of the almost hopeless contradictions of the different systems, we find the golden thread of unity running through them all, and in this philosophy, this golden thread has been traced revealed little by little to our view, and the first step to this revelation is the common ground that all are advancing towards freedom.

One curious fact present in the midst of all our joys and sorrows, difficulties and struggles, is that we are surely journeying towards freedom. The question was practically this: "What is this universe? From what does it arise? Into what does it go?" And the answer was: "In freedom it rises, in freedom it rests, and into freedom it melts away." This idea of freedom you cannot relinquish. Your actions, your very lives will be lost without it. Every moment nature is proving us to be slaves and not free. Yet, simultaneously rises the other idea, that still we are free At every step we are knocked down, as it were, by Maya, and shown that we are bound; and yet at the same moment, together with this blow, together with this feeling that we are bound, comes the other feeling that we are free. Some inner voice tells us that we are free. But if we attempt to realise that freedom, to make it manifest, we find the difficulties almost insuperable Yet, in spite of that it insists on asserting itself inwardly, "I am free, I am free." And if you study all the various religions of the world you will find this idea expressed. Not only religion – you must not take this word in its narrow sense – but the whole life of society is the assertion of that one principle of freedom. All movements are the assertion of that one freedom. That voice has been heard by everyone, whether he knows it or not, that voice which declares, "Come unto Me all ye that labour and are heavy laden." It may not be in the same language or the same form of speech, but in some form or other, that voice calling for freedom has been with us. Yes, we are born here on account of that voice; every one of our movements is for that. We are all rushing towards freedom, we are all following that voice, whether we know it or not; as the children of the village were attracted by the music of the flute-player, so we are all following the music of the voice without knowing it.

We are ethical when we follow that voice. Not only the human soul, but all creatures, from the lowest to the highest have heard the voice and are rushing towards it; and in the struggle are either combining with each other or pushing each other out of the way. Thus come competition, joys, struggles, life, pleasure, and death, and the whole universe is nothing but the result of this mad struggle to reach the voice. This is the manifestation of nature.

What happens then? The scene begins to shift. As soon as you know the voice and understand what it is, the whole scene changes. The same world which was the ghastly battle-field of Maya is now changed into something good and beautiful. We no longer curse nature, nor say that the world is horrible and that it is all vain; we need no longer weep and wail. As soon as we understand the voice, we see the reassert why this struggle should be here, this fight, this competition, this difficulty, this cruelty, these little pleasures and joys; we see that they are in the nature of things, because without them there would be no going towards the voice, to attain which we are destined, whether we know it or not. All human life, all nature, therefore, is struggling to attain to freedom. The sun is moving towards the goal, so is the earth in circling round the sun, so is the moon in circling round the earth. To that goal the planet is moving, and the air is blowing. Everything is struggling towards that. The saint is going towards that voice — he cannot help it, it is no glory to him. So is the sinner. The charitable man is going straight towards that voice, and cannot be hindered; the miser is also going towards the same destination: the greatest worker of good hears the same voice within, and he cannot resist it, he must go towards the voice; so with the most arrant idler. One stumbles more than another, and him who stumbles more we call bad, him who stumbles less we call good. Good and bad are never two different things, they are one and the same; the difference is not one of kind, but of degree.

Now, if the manifestation of this power of freedom is really governing the whole universe — applying that to religion, our special study — we find this idea has been the one assertion throughout. Take the lowest form of religion where there is the worship of departed ancestors or certain powerful and cruel gods; what is the prominent idea about the gods or departed ancestors? That they are superior to nature, not bound by its restrictions. The worshipper has, no doubt, very limited ideas of nature. He himself cannot pass through a wall, nor fly up into the skies, but the gods whom he worships can do these things. What is meant by that, philosophically? That the assertion of freedom is there, that the gods whom he worships are superior to nature as he knows it. So with those who worship still higher beings. As the idea of nature expands, the idea of the soul which is superior to nature also expands, until we come to what we call monotheism, which holds that there is Maya (nature), and that there is some Being who is the Ruler of this Maya.

Here Vedanta begins, where these monotheistic ideas first appear. But the Vedanta philosophy wants further explanation. This explanation — that there is a Being beyond all these manifestations of Maya, who is superior to and independent of Maya, and who is attracting us towards Himself, and that we are all going towards Him — is very good, says the Vedanta, but yet the perception is not clear, the vision is dim and hazy, although it does not directly contradict reason. Just as in your hymn it is said, "Nearer my God to Thee," the same hymn would be very good to the Vedantin, only he would change a word, and make it, "Nearer my God to me." The idea that the goal is far off, far beyond nature, attracting us all towards it, has to be brought nearer and nearer, without degrading or degenerating it. The God of heaven becomes the God in nature, and the God in nature becomes the God who is nature, and the God who is nature becomes the God within this temple of the body, and the God dwelling in the temple of the body at last becomes the temple itself, becomes the soul and man – and there it reaches the last words it can teach. He whom the sages have been seeking in all these places is in our own hearts; the voice that you heard was right, says the Vedanta, but the direction you gave to the voice was wrong. That ideal of freedom that you perceived was correct, but you projected it outside yourself, and that was your mistake. Bring it nearer and nearer, until you find that it was all the time within you, it was the Self of your own self. That freedom was your own nature, and this Maya never bound you. Nature never has power over you. Like a frightened child you were dreaming that it was throttling you, and the release from this fear is the goal: not only to see it intellectually, but to perceive it, actualise it, much more definitely than we perceive this world. Then we shall know that we are free. Then, and then alone, will all difficulties vanish, then will all the perplexities of heart be smoothed away, all crookedness made straight, then will vanish the delusion of manifoldness and nature; and Maya instead of being a horrible, hopeless dream, as it is now will become beautiful, and this earth, instead of being a prison-house, will become our playground, and even dangers and difficulties, even all sufferings, will become deified and show us their real nature, will show us that behind everything, as the substance of everything, He is standing, and that He is the one real Self.

❑

6

The Absolute and Manifestation

(Delivered in London, 1896)

The one question that is most difficult to grasp in understanding the Advaita philosophy, and the one question that will be asked again and again and that will always remain is: How has the Infinite, the Absolute, become the finite? I will now take up this question, and, in order to illustrate it, I will use a figure.

Here is the Absolute (a), and this is the universe (b). The Absolute has become the universe.By this is not only meant the material world, but the mental world, the spiritual world – heavens and earths, and in fact, everything that exists. Mind is the name of a change, and body the name of another change, and so on, and all these changes compose our universe. This Absolute (a) has become the universe (b) by coming through time, space, and causation (c). This is the central idea of Advaita. Time, space, and causation are like the glass through which the Absolute is seen, and when It is seen on the lower side, It appears as the universe. Now we at once gather from this that in the Absolute there is neither time, space, nor causation. The idea of time cannot be there, seeing that there is no mind, no thought. The idea of space cannot be there, seeing that there is no external change. What you call motion and causation cannot exist where there is only One. We have to understand this, and impress

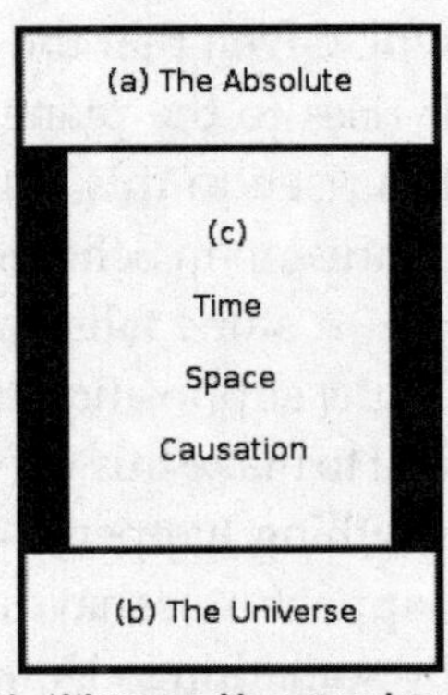

it on our minds, that what we call causation begins after, if we may be permitted to say so, the degeneration of the Absolute into the phenomenal, and not before; that our will, our desire and all these things always come after that. I think Schopenhauer's philosophy makes a mistake in its interpretation of Vedanta, for it seeks to make the will everything. Schopenhauer makes the will stand in the place of the Absolute. But the absolute cannot be presented as will, for will is something changeable and phenomenal, and over the line, drawn above time, space, and causation, there is no change, no motion; it is only below the line that external motion and internal motion, called thought begin. There can be no will on the other side, and will therefore, cannot be the cause of this universe. Coming nearer, we see in our own bodies that will is not the cause of every movement. I move this chair; my will is the cause of this movement, and this will becomes manifested as muscular motion at the other end. But the same power that moves the chair is moving the heart, the lungs, and so on, but not through will. Given that the power is the same, it only becomes will when it rises to the plane of consciousness, and to call it will before it has risen to this plane is a misnomer. This makes a good deal of confusion in Schopenhauer's philosophy.

A stone falls and we ask, why? This question is possible only on the supposition that nothing happens without a cause. I request you to make this very clear in your minds, for whenever we ask why anything happens, we are taking for granted that everything that happens must have a why, that is to say, it must have been preceded by something else which acted as the cause. This precedence and succession are what we call the law of causation. It means that everything in the universe is by turn a cause and an effect. It is the cause of certain things which come after it, and is itself the effect of something else which has preceded it. This is called the law of causation and is a necessary condition of all our thinking. We believe that every particle in the universe, whatever it be, is in relation to every other particle. There has been much discussion as to how this idea arose. In Europe, there have been intuitive philosophers who believed that it was constitutional in humanity, others have believed it came from experience, but the question has never been settled. We shall see later on what the Vedanta has to say about it. But first we have to understand this that the very asking of the question "why" presupposes that everything round us has been preceded by certain things and will be succeeded by certain other things. The other belief involved in this question is that nothing in the universe is independent, that everything is acted upon by something outside itself. Interdependence is the law of the whole universe. In asking what caused the Absolute, what an error we are making! To ask this question we have to suppose that the Absolute also is bound by something, that It is dependent on something; and in making this supposition, we drag the Absolute down to the level of the universe. For in the Absolute there is neither time, space, nor causation; It is all one. That which exists by itself alone cannot have any cause. That which is free cannot have any cause; else it would not be free, but bound. That which has relativity cannot be free. Thus we see the very question, why the Infinite became the finite, is an impossible one, for it is self-contradictory. Coming from subtleties to the logic of our common plane, to common sense, we can see this from another side, when we seek to know how the Absolute has become the relative. Supposing we knew the answer, would the Absolute remain the Absolute? It would have become relative. What is meant by knowledge in our common-sense idea? It is only something that has become limited by our mind, that we know, and when it is beyond our mind, it is not knowledge. Now if the Absolute becomes limited by the mind, It is no more Absolute; It has become finite. Everything limited by the mind becomes finite. Therefore to know the Absolute is again a contradiction in terms. That is why this question has never been answered, because if it were answered, there would no more be an Absolute. A God known is no more God; He has become finite like one of us. He cannot be known He is always the Unknowable One.

But what Advaita says is that God is more than knowable. This is a great fact to learn. You must not go home with the idea that God is unknowable in the sense in which agnostics put it. For instance, here is a chair, it is known to us. But what is beyond ether or whether people exist there or not is possibly unknowable. But God is neither known nor unknowable in this sense. He is something still higher than known; that is what is meant by God being unknown and unknowable. The expression is not used in the sense in which it may be said that some questions are unknown ant unknowable. God is more than known. This chair is known, but God is intensely more than that because in and through Him we have to know this chair itself. He is the Witness, the eternal Witness of all knowledge. Whatever we know we have to know in and through Him. He is the Essence of our own Self. He is the Essence of this ego, this I and we cannot know anything excepting in and through that I. Therefore you have to know everything in and through the Brahman. To know the chair you have to know it in and through God. Thus God is infinitely nearer to us than the chair, but yet He is infinitely higher. Neither known, nor unknown, but something infinitely higher than either. He is your Self. "Who would live a second, who would breathe a second in this universe, if that Blessed One were not filling it?" Because in and through Him we breathe, in and through Him we exist. Not the He is standing somewhere and making my blood circulate. What is meant is that He is the Essence of all this, tie Soul of my soul. You cannot by any possibility say you know Him; it would be degrading Him. You cannot get out of yourself, so you cannot know Him. Knowledge is objectification. For instance, in memory you are objectifying many things, projecting them out of yourself. All memory, all the things which I have seen and which I know are in my mind. The pictures, the impressions of all these things, are in my mind, and when I would try to think of them, to know them, the first act of knowledge would be to project them outside. This cannot be done with God, because He is the Essence of our souls, we cannot project Him outside ourselves. Here is one of the profoundest passages in Vedanta: "He that is the Essence of your soul, He is the Truth, He is the Self, thou art That, O Shvetaketu." This is what is meant by "Thou art God." You cannot describe Him by any other language. All attempts of language, calling Him father, or brother, or our dearest friend, are attempts to objectify

God, which cannot be done. He is the Eternal Subject of everything. I am the subject of this chair; I see the chair; so God is the Eternal Subject of my soul. How can you objectify Him, the Essence of your souls, the Reality of everything? Thus, I would repeat to you once more, God is neither knowable nor unknowable, but something infinitely higher than either. He is one with us, and that which is one with us is neither knowable nor unknowable, as our own self. You cannot know your own self; you cannot move it out and make it an object to look at, because you are that and cannot separate yourself from it. Neither is it unknowable, for what is better known than yourself? It is really the centre of our knowledge. In exactly the same sense, God is neither unknowable nor known, but infinitely higher than both; for He is our real Self.

First, we see then that the question, "What caused the Absolute?" is a contradiction in terms; and secondly, we find that the idea of God in the Advaita is this Oneness; and, therefore, we cannot objectify Him, for we are always living and moving in Him, whether we know it or not. Whatever we do is always through Him. Now the question is: What are time, space, and causation? Advaita means non-duality; there are no two, but one. Yet we see that here is a proposition that the Absolute is manifesting Itself as many, through the veil of time, space, and causation. Therefore it seems that here are two, the Absolute and Mâyâ (the sum total of time, space, and causation). It seems apparently very convincing that there are two. To this the Advaitist replies that it cannot be called two. To have two, we must have two absolute independent existences which cannot be caused. In the first place time, space, and causation cannot be said to be independent existences. Time is entirely a dependent existence; it changes with every change of our mind. Sometimes in dream one imagines that one has lived several years, at other times several months were passed as one second. So, time is entirely dependent on our state of mind. Secondly, the idea of time vanishes altogether, sometimes. So with space. We cannot know what space is. Yet it is there, indefinable, and cannot exist separate from anything else. So with causation.

The one peculiar attribute we find in time, space, and causation is that they cannot exist separate from other things. Try to think of space without colour, or limits, or any connection with the things around — just abstract space. You cannot; you have to think of it as the space between two limits or between three objects. It has to be connected with some object to have any existence. So with time; you cannot have any idea of abstract time, but you have to take two events, one preceding and the other succeeding, and join the two events by the idea of succession. Time depends on two events, just as space has to be related to outside objects. And the idea of causation is inseparable from time and space. This is the peculiar thing about them that they have no independent existence. They have not even the existence which the chair or the wall has. They are as shadows around everything which you cannot catch. They have no real existence; yet they are not non-existent, seeing that through them all things are manifesting as this universe. Thus we see, first, that the combination of time, space, and causation has neither existence nor non-existence. Secondly, it sometimes vanishes. To give an illustration, there is a wave on the ocean. The wave is the same as the ocean certainly, and yet we know it is a wave, and as such different from the ocean. What makes this difference? The name and the form, that is, the idea in the mind and the form. Now, can we think of a wave-form as something separate from the ocean? Certainly not. It is always associated with the ocean idea. If the wave subsides, the form vanishes in a moment, and yet the form was not a delusion. So long as the wave existed the form was there, and you were bound to see the form. This is Maya.

The whole of this universe, therefore, is, as it were, a peculiar form; the Absolute is that ocean while you and I, and suns and stars, and everything else are various waves of that ocean. And what makes the waves different? Only the form, and that form is time, space, and causation, all entirely dependent on the wave. As soon as the wave goes, they vanish. As soon as the individual gives up this Maya, it vanishes for him and he becomes free. The whole struggle is to get rid of this clinging on to time, space, and causation, which are always obstacles in our way. What is the theory of evolution? What are the two factors? A tremendous potential power which is trying to express itself, and circumstances which are holding it down, the environments not allowing it to express itself. So, in order to fight with these environments, the power is taking new bodies again and again. An amoeba, in the struggle, gets another body and conquers some obstacles, then gets another body and so on, until it becomes man. Now, if you carry this idea to its logical conclusion, there must come a time when that power that was in the amoeba and which evolved as man will have conquered all the obstructions that nature can bring before it and will thus escape from all its environments. This idea expressed in metaphysics will take this form; there are two components in every action, the one the subject, the other the object and the one aim of life is to make the subject master of the object. For instance, I feel unhappy because a man scolds me. My struggle will be to make myself strong enough to conquer the environment, so that he may scold and I shall not feel. That is how we are all trying to conquer. What is meant by morality? Making the subject strong by attuning it to the Absolute, so that finite nature ceases to have control over us. It is a logical conclusion of our philosophy that there must come a time when we shall have conquered all the environments, because nature is finite.

Here is another thing to learn. How do you know that nature is finite? You can only know this through metaphysics. Nature is that Infinite under limitations. Therefore it is finite. So, there must come a time when we shall have conquered all environments. And how are we to conquer them? We cannot possibly conquer all the objective environments. We cannot. The little fish wants to fly from its enemies in the water. How does it do so? By evolving wings and becoming a bird. The fish did not change the water or the air; the change was in itself. Change is always subjective. All through evolution you find that the conquest of nature comes by change in the subject. Apply this to religion and morality, and you will find that the conquest of evil comes by the change in the subjective alone. That is how the Advaita system gets its whole force, on the subjective side of man. To talk of evil and misery is nonsense, because they do not exist outside. If I am immune against all anger, I never feel angry. If I am proof against all hatred, I never feel hatred.

This is, therefore, the process by which to achieve that conquest — through the subjective, by perfecting the subjective. I may make bold to say that the only religion which agrees with, and even goes a little further than modern researches, both on physical and moral lines is the Advaita, and that is why it appeals to modern scientists so much. They find that the old dualistic theories are not enough for them, do not satisfy their necessities. A man must have not only faith, but intellectual faith too. Now, in this later part of the nineteenth century, such an idea as that religion coming from any other source than one's own hereditary religion must be false shows that there is still weakness left, and such ideas must be given up. I do not mean that such is the case in this country alone, it is in every country, and nowhere more than in my own. This Advaita was never allowed to come to the people. At first some monks got hold of it and took it to the forests, and so it came to be called the "Forest Philosophy". By the mercy of the Lord, the Buddha came and preached it to the masses, and the whole nation became Buddhists. Long after that, when atheists and agnostics had destroyed the nation again, it was found out that Advaita was the only way to save India from materialism.

Thus has Advaita twice saved India from materialism Before the Buddha came, materialism had spread to a fearful extent, and it was of a most hideous kind, not like that of the present day, but of a far worse nature. I am a materialist in a certain sense, because I believe that there is only One. That is what the materialist wants you to believe; only he calls it matter and I call it God. The materialists admit that out of this matter all hope, and religion, and everything have come. I say, all these have come out of Brahman. But the materialism that prevailed before Buddha was that crude sort of materialism which taught, "Eat, drink, and be merry; there is no God, soul or heaven; religion is a concoction of wicked priests." It taught the morality that so long as you live, you must try to live happily; eat, though you have to borrow money for the food, and never mind about repaying it. That was the old materialism, and that kind of philosophy spread so much that even today it has got the name of "popular philosophy". Buddha brought the Vedanta to light, gave it to the people, and saved India. A thousand years after his death a similar state of things again prevailed. The mobs, the masses, and various races, had been converted to Buddhism; naturally the teachings of the Buddha became in time degenerated, because most of the people were very ignorant. Buddhism taught no God, no Ruler of the universe, so gradually the masses brought their gods, and devils, and hobgoblins out again, and a tremendous hotchpotch was made of Buddhism in India. Again materialism came to the fore, taking the form of licence with the higher classes and superstition with the lower. Then Shankaracharya arose and once more revivified the Vedanta philosophy. He made it a rationalistic philosophy. In the Upanishads the arguments are often very obscure. By Buddha the moral side of the philosophy was laid stress upon, and by Shankaracharya, the intellectual side. He worked out, rationalised, and placed before men the wonderful coherent system of Advaita.

Materialism prevails in Europe today. You may pray for the salvation of the modern sceptics, but they do not yield, they want reason. The salvation of Europe depends on a rationalistic religion, and Advaita — the non-duality, the Oneness, the idea of the Impersonal God — is the only religion that can have any hold on any intellectual people. It comes whenever religion seems to disappear and irreligion seems to prevail, and that is why it has taken ground in Europe and America.

I would say one thing more in connection with this philosophy. In the old Upanishads we find sublime poetry; their authors were poets. Plato says, inspiration comes to people through poetry, and it seems as if these ancient Rishis, seers of Truth, were raised above humanity to show these truths through poetry. They never preached, nor philosophised, nor wrote. Music came out of their hearts. In Buddha we had the great, universal heart and infinite patience, making religion practical and bringing it to everyone's door. In Shankaracharya we saw tremendous intellectual power, throwing the scorching light of reason upon everything. We want today that bright sun of intellectuality joined with the heart of Buddha, the wonderful infinite heart of love and mercy. This union will give us the highest philosophy. Science and religion will meet and shake hands. Poetry and philosophy will become friends. This will be the religion of the future, and if we can work it out, we may be sure that it will be for all times and peoples. This is the one way that will prove acceptable to modern science, for it has almost come to it. When the scientific teacher asserts that all things are the manifestation of one force, does it not remind you of the God of whom you hear in the Upanishads: "As the one fire entering into the universe expresses itself in various forms, even so that One Soul is expressing Itself in every soul and yet is infinitely more besides?" Do you not see whither science is tending? The Hindu nation proceeded through the study of the mind, through metaphysics and logic. The European nations start from external nature, and now they too are coming to the same results. We find that searching through the mind we at last come to that Oneness, that Universal One, the Internal Soul of everything, the Essence and Reality of everything, the Ever-Free, the Ever-blissful, the Ever-Existing. Through material science we come to the same Oneness. Science today is telling us that all things are but the manifestation of one energy which is the sum total of everything which exists, and the trend of humanity is towards freedom and not towards bondage. Why should men be moral? Because through morality is the path towards freedom, and immorality leads to bondage.

Another peculiarity of the Advaita system is that from its very start it is non-destructive. This is another glory, the boldness to preach, "Do not disturb the faith of any, even of those who through ignorance have attached themselves to lower forms of worship." That is what it says, do not disturb, but help everyone to get higher and higher; include all humanity. This philosophy preaches a God who is a sum total. If you seek a universal religion which can apply to everyone, that religion must not be composed of only the parts, but it must always be their sum total and include all degrees of religious development.

This idea is not clearly found in any other religious system. They are all parts equally struggling to attain to the whole. The existence of the part is only for this. So, from the very first, Advaita had no antagonism with the various sects existing in India. There are dualists existing today, and their number is by far the largest in India, because dualism naturally appeals to less educated minds. It is a very convenient, natural, common-sense explanation of the universe. But with these dualists, Advaita has no quarrel. The one thinks that God is outside the universe, somewhere in heaven, and the other, that He is his own Soul, and that it will be a blasphemy to call Him anything more distant. Any idea of separation would be terrible. He is the nearest of the near. There is no word in any language to express this nearness except the word Oneness. With any other idea the Advaitist is not satisfied just as the dualist is shocked with the concept of the Advaita, and thinks it blasphemous. At the same time the Advaitist knows that these other ideas must be, and so has no quarrel with the dualist who is on the right road. From his standpoint, the dualist will have to see many. It is a constitutional necessity of his standpoint. Let him have it. The Advaitist knows that whatever may be his theories, he is going to the same goal as he himself. There he differs entirely from dualist who is forced by his point of view to believe that all differing views are wrong. The dualists all the world over naturally believe in a Personal God who is purely anthropomorphic, who like a great potentate in this world is pleased with some and displeased with others. He is arbitrarily pleased with some people or races and showers blessing upon them. Naturally the dualist comes to the conclusion that God has favourites, and he hopes to be one of them. You will find that in almost every religion is the idea: "We are the favourites of our God, and only by believing as we do, can you be taken into favour with Him." Some dualists are so narrow as to insist that only the few that have been predestined to the favour of God can be saved; the rest may try ever so hard, but they cannot be accepted. I challenge you to show me one dualistic religion which has not more or less of this exclusiveness. And, therefore, in the nature of things, dualistic religions are bound to fight and quarrel with each other, and this they have ever been doing. Again, these dualists win the popular favour by appealing to the vanity of the uneducated. They like to feel that they enjoy exclusive privileges. The dualist thinks you cannot be moral until you have a God with a rod in His hand, ready to punish you. The unthinking masses are generally dualists, and they, poor fellows, have been persecuted for thousands of years in every country; and their idea of salvation is, therefore, freedom from the fear of punishment. I was asked by a clergyman in America, "What! you have no Devil in your religion? How can that be?" But we find that the best and the greatest men that have been born in the world have worked with that high impersonal idea. It is the Man who said, "I and my Father are One", whose power has descended unto millions. For thousands of years it has worked for good. And we know that the same Man, because he was a nondualist, was merciful to others. To the masses who could not conceive of anything higher than a Personal God, he said, "Pray to your Father in heaven." To others who could grasp a higher idea, he said, "I am the vine, ye are the branches," but to his disciples to whom he revealed himself more fully, he proclaimed the highest truth, "I and my Father are One."

It was the great Buddha, who never cared for the dualist gods, and who has been called an atheist and materialist, who yet was ready to give up his body for a poor goat. That Man set in motion the highest moral ideas any nation can have. Whenever there is a moral code, it is ray of light from that Man. We cannot force the great hearts of the world into narrow limits, and keep them there, especially at this time in the history of humanity when there is a degree of intellectual development such as was never dreamed of even a hundred years ago, when a wave of scientific knowledge has arisen which nobody, even fifty years ago, would have dreamed of. By trying to force people into narrow limits you degrade them into animals and unthinking masses. You kill their moral life. What is now wanted is a combination of the greatest heart with the highest intellectuality, of infinite love with infinite knowledge. The Vedantist gives no other attributes to God except these three – that He is Infinite Existence, Infinite Knowledge, and Infinite Bliss, and he regards these three as One. Existence without knowledge and love cannot be; knowledge without love and love without knowledge cannot be. What we want is the harmony of Existence, Knowledge, and Bliss Infinite. For that is our goal. We want harmony, not one-sided development. And it is possible to have the intellect of a Shankara with the heart of a Buddha. I hope we shall all struggle to attain to that blessed combination.

❑

7

God in Everything

(Delivered in London, 27th October 1896)

We have seen how the greater portion of our life must of necessity be filled with evils, however we may resist, and that this mass of evil is practically almost infinite for us. We have been struggling to remedy this since the beginning of time, yet everything remains very much the same. The more we discover remedies, the more we find ourselves beset by subtler evils. We have also seen that all religions propose a God, as the one way of escaping these difficulties. All religions tell us that if you take the world as it is, as most practical people would advise us to do in this age, then nothing would be left to us but evil. They further assert that there is something beyond this world. This life in the five senses, life in the material world, is not all; it is only a small portion, and merely superficial. Behind and beyond is the Infinite in which there is no more evil. Some people call It God, some Allah, some Jehovah, Jove, and so on. The Vedantin calls It Brahman.

The first impression we get of the advice given by religions is that we had better terminate our existence. To the question how to cure the evils of life, the answer apparently is, give up life. It reminds one of the old story. A mosquito settled on the head of a man, and a friend, wishing to kill the mosquito, gave it such a blow that he killed both man and mosquito. The remedy of evil seems to suggest a similar course of action. Life is full of ills, the world is full of evils; that is a fact no one who is old enough to know the world can deny.

But what is remedy proposed by all the religions? That this world is nothing. Beyond this world is something which is very real. Here comes the difficulty. The remedy seems to destroy everything. How can that be a remedy? Is there no way out then? The Vedanta says that what all the religions advance is perfectly true, but it should be properly understood. Often it is misunderstood, because the religions are not very clear in their meaning. What we really want is head and heart combined. The heart is great indeed; it is through the heart that come the great inspirations of life. I would a hundred times rather have a little heart and no brain, than be all brains and no heart. Life is possible, progress is possible for him who has heart, but he who has no heart and only brains dies of dryness.

At the same time we know that he who is carried along by his heart alone has to undergo many ills, for now and then he is liable to tumble into pitfalls. The combination of heart and head is what we want. I do not mean that a man should compromise his heart for his brain or vice versa, but let everyone have an infinite amount of heart and feeling, and at the same time an infinite amount of reason. Is there any limit to what we want in this world? Is not the world infinite? There is room for an infinite amount of feeling, and so also for an infinite amount of culture and reason. Let them come together without limit, let them be running together, as it were, in parallel lines each with the other.

Most of the religions understand the fact, but the error into which they all seem to fall is the same; they are carried away by the heart, the feelings. There is evil in the world, give up the world; that is the great teaching, and the only teaching, no doubt. Give up the world. There cannot be two opinions that to understand the truth everyone of us has to give up error. There cannot be two opinions that everyone of us in order to have good must give up evil; there cannot be two opinions that everyone of us to have life must give up what is death.

And yet, what remains to us, if this theory involves giving up the life of the senses, the life as we know it? And what else do we mean by life? If we give this up, what remains?

We shall understand this better, when, later on, we come to the more philosophical portions of the Vedanta. But for the present I beg to state that in Vedanta alone we find a rational solution of the problem. Here I can only lay before you what the Vedanta seeks to teach, and that is the deification of the world. The Vedanta does not in reality denounce the world. The ideal of renunciation nowhere attains such a height as in the teachings of the Vedanta. But, at the same time, dry suicidal advice is not intended; it really means deification of the world – giving up the world as we think of it, as we know it, as it appears to us – and to know what it really is. Deify it; it is God alone. We read at the commencement of one of the oldest of the Upanishads, "Whatever exists in this universe is to be covered with the Lord."

We have to cover everything with the Lord Himself, not by a false sort of optimism, not by blinding our eyes to the evil, but by really seeing God in everything. Thus we have to give up the world, and when the world is given up, what remains? God. What is meant? You can have your wife; it does not mean that you are to abandon her, but that you are to see God in the wife. Give up your children; what does that mean? To turn them out of doors, as some human brutes do in every country? Certainly not. That is diabolism; it is not religion. But see God in your children. So, in everything. In life and in death, in happiness and in misery, the Lord is equally present. The whole world is full of the Lord. Open your eyes and see Him. This is what Vedanta teaches. Give up the world which you have conjectured, because your conjecture was based upon a very partial experience, upon very poor reasoning, and upon your own weakness. Give it up; the world we have been thinking of so long, the world to which we have been clinging so long, is a false world of our own creation. Give that up; open your eyes and see that as such it never existed; it was a dream, Maya. What existed was the Lord Himself. It is He who is in the child, in the wife, and in the husband; it is He who is in the good and in the bad; He is in the sin and in the sinner; He is in life and in death.

A tremendous assertion indeed! Yet that is the theme which the Vedanta wants to demonstrate, to teach, and to preach. This is just the opening theme.

Thus we avoid the dangers of life and its evils. Do not desire anything. What makes us miserable? The cause of all miseries from which we suffer is desire. You desire something, and the desire is not fulfilled; the result is distress. If there is no desire, there is no suffering. But here, too, there is the danger of my being misunderstood. So it is necessary to explain what I mean by giving up desire and becoming free from all misery. The walls have no desire and they never suffer. True, but they never evolve. This chair has no desires, it never suffers; but it is always a chair. There is a glory in happiness, there is a glory in suffering. If I may dare to say so, there is a utility in evil too. The great lesson in misery we all know. There are hundreds of things we have done in our lives which we wish we had never done, but which, at the same time, have been great teachers. As for me, I am glad I have done something good and many things bad; glad I have done something right, and glad I have committed many errors, because every one of them has been a great lesson. I, as I am now, am the resultant of all I have done, all I have thought. Every action and thought have had their effect, and these effects are the sum total of my progress.

We all understand that desires are wrong, but what is meant by giving up desires? How could life go on? It would be the same suicidal advice, killing the desire and the man too. The solution is this. Not that you should not have property, not that you should not have things which are necessary and things which are even luxuries. Have all that you want, and more, only know the truth and realise it. Wealth does not belong to anybody. Have no idea of proprietorship, possessorship. You are nobody, nor am I, nor anyone else. All belongs to the Lord, because the opening verse told us to put the Lord in everything.

God is in the wealth that you enjoy. He is in the desire that rises in your mind. He is in the things you buy to satisfy your desire; He is in your beautiful attire, in your beautiful ornaments. This is the line of thought. All will be metamorphosed as soon as you begin to see things in that light. If you put God in your every movement, in your conversation, in your form, in everything, the whole scene changes, and the world, instead of appearing as one of woe and misery, will become a heaven.

"The kingdom of heaven is within you," says Jesus; so says the Vedanta, and every great teacher. "He that hath eyes to see, let him see, and he that hath ears to hear, let him hear." The Vedanta proves that the truth for which we have been searching all this time is present, and was all the time with us. In our ignorance, we thought we had lost it, and went about the world crying and weeping, struggling to find the truth, while all along it was dwelling in our own hearts. There alone can we find it.

If we understand the giving up of the world in its old, crude sense, then it would come to this: that we must not work, that we must be idle, sitting like lumps of earth, neither thinking nor doing anything, but must become fatalists, driven about by every circumstance, ordered about by the laws of nature, drifting from place to place. That would be the result. But that is not what is meant. We must work. Ordinary mankind, driven everywhere by false desire, what do they know of work? The man propelled by his own feelings and his own senses, what does he know about work? He works, who is not propelled by his own desires, by any selfishness whatsoever. He works, who has no ulterior motive in view. He works, who has nothing to gain from work.

Who enjoys the picture, the seller or the seer? The seller is busy with his accounts, computing what his gain will be, how much profit he will realise on the picture. His brain is full of that. He is looking at the hammer, and watching the bids. He is intent on hearing how fast the bids are rising. That man is enjoying the picture who has gone there without any intention of buying or selling. He looks at the picture and enjoys it. So this whole universe is a picture, and when these desires have vanished, men will enjoy the world, and then this buying and selling and these foolish ideas of possession will be ended. The money-lender gone, the buyer gone, the seller gone, this world remains the picture, a beautiful painting. I never read of any more beautiful conception of God than the following: "He is the Great Poet, the Ancient Poet; the whole universe is His poem, coming in verses and rhymes and rhythms, written in infinite bliss." When we have given up desires, then alone shall we be able to read and enjoy this universe of God. Then everything will become deified. Nooks and corners, by-ways and shady places, which we thought dark and unholy, will be all deified. They will all reveal their true nature, and we shall smile at ourselves and think that all this weeping and crying has been but child's play, and we were only standing by, watching.

So, do your work, says the Vedanta. It first advises us how to work – by giving up – giving up the apparent, illusive world. What is meant by that? Seeing God everywhere. Thus do you work. Desire to live a hundred years, have all earthly desires, if you wish, only deify them, convert them into heaven. Have the desire to live a long life of helpfulness, of blissfulness and activity on this earth. Thus working, you will find the way out. There is no other way. If a man plunges headlong into foolish luxuries of the world without knowing the truth, he has missed his footing, he cannot reach the goal. And if a man curses the world, goes into a forest, mortifies his flesh, and kills himself little by little by starvation, makes his heart a barren waste, kills out all feelings, and becomes harsh, stern, and dried-up, that man also has missed the way. These are the two extremes, the two mistakes at either end. Both have lost the way, both have missed the goal.

So work, says the Vedanta, putting God in everything, and knowing Him to be in everything. Work incessantly, holding life as something deified, as God Himself, and knowing that this is all we have to do, this is all we should ask for. God is in everything, where else shall we go to find Him? He is already in every work, in every thought, in every feeling. Thus knowing, we must work — this is the only way, there is no other. Thus the effects of work will not bind us. We have seen how false desires are the cause of all the misery and evil we suffer, but when they are thus deified, purified, through God, they bring no evil, they bring no misery. Those who have not learnt this secret will have to live in a demoniacal world until they discover it. Many do not know what an infinite mine of bliss is in them, around them, everywhere; they have not yet discovered it. What is a demoniacal world? The Vedanta says, ignorance.

We are dying of thirst sitting on the banks of the mightiest river. We are dying of hunger sitting near heaps of food. Here is the blissful universe, yet we do not find it. We are in it all the time, and we are always mistaking it. Religion proposes to find this out for us. The longing for this blissful universe is in all hearts. It has been the search of all nations, it is the one goal of religion, and this ideal is expressed in various languages in different religions. It is only the difference of language that makes all these apparent divergences. One expresses a thought in one way, another a little differently, yet perhaps each is meaning exactly what the other is expressing in a different language.

More questions arise in connection with this. It is very easy to talk. From my childhood I have heard of seeing God everywhere and in everything, and then I can really enjoy the world, but as soon as I mix with the world, and get a few blows from it, the idea vanishes. I am walking in the street thinking that God is in every man, and a strong man comes along and gives me a push and I fall flat on the footpath. Then I rise up quickly with clenched fist, the blood has rushed to my head, and the reflection goes. Immediately I have become mad. Everything is forgotten; instead of encountering God I see the devil. Ever since we were born we have been told to see God in all. Every religion teaches that — see God in everything and everywhere. Do you not remember in the New Testament how Christ says so? We have all been taught that; but it is when we come to the practical side, that the difficulty begins. You all remember how in *Æesop's Fables* a fine stag is looking at his form reflected in a lake and is saying to his young one, "How powerful I am, look at my splendid head, look at my limbs, how strong and muscular they are; and how swiftly I can run." In the meantime he hears the barking of dogs in the distance, and immediately takes to his heels, and after he has run several miles, he comes back panting. The young one says, "You just told me how strong you were, how was it that when the dog barked, you ran away?" "Yes, my son; but when the dogs bark all my confidence vanishes." Such is the case with us. We think highly of humanity, we feel ourselves strong and valiant, we make grand resolves; but when the "dogs" of trial and temptation bark, we are like the stag in the fable. Then, if such is the case, what is the use of teaching all these things? There is the greatest use. The use is this, that perseverance will finally conquer. Nothing can be done in a day.

"This Self is first to be heard, then to be thought upon, and then meditated upon." Everyone can see the sky, even the very worm crawling upon the earth sees the blue sky, but how very far away it is! So it is with our ideal. It is far away, no doubt, but at the same time, we know that we must have it. We must even have the highest ideal. Unfortunately in this life, the vast majority of persons are groping through this dark life without any ideal at all. If a man with an ideal makes a thousand mistakes, I am sure that the man without an ideal makes fifty thousand. Therefore, it is better to have an ideal. And this ideal we must hear about as much as we can, till it enters into our hearts, into our brains, into our very veins, until it tingles in every drop of our blood and permeates every pore in our body. We must meditate upon it. "Out of the fullness of the heart the mouth speaketh," and out of the fullness of the heart the hand works too.

It is thought which is the propelling force in us. Fill the mind with the highest thoughts, hear them day after day, think them month after month. Never mind failures; they are quite natural, they are the beauty of life, these failures. What would life be without them? It would not be worth having if it were not for struggles. Where would be the poetry of life? Never mind the struggles, the mistakes. I never heard a cow tell a lie, but it is only a cow – never a man. So never mind these failures, these little backslidings; hold the ideal a thousand times, and if you fail a thousand times, make the attempt once more. The ideal of man is to see God in everything. But if you cannot see Him in everything, see Him in one thing, in that thing which you like best, and then see Him in another. So on you can go. There is infinite life before the soul. Take your time and you will achieve your end.

"He, the One, who vibrates more quickly than mind, who attains to more speed than mind can ever do, whom even the gods reach not, nor thought grasps, He moving, everything moves. In Him all exists. He is moving. He is also immovable. He is near and He is far. He is inside everything. He is outside everything, interpenetrating everything. Whoever sees in every being that same Atman, and whoever sees everything in that Atman, he never goes far from that Atman. When all life and the whole universe are seen in this Atman, then alone man has attained the secret. There is no more delusion for him. Where is any more misery for him who sees this Oneness in the universe?"

This is another great theme of the Vedanta, this Oneness of life, this Oneness of everything. We shall see how it demonstrates that all our misery comes through ignorance, and this ignorance is the idea of manifoldness, this separation between man and man, between nation and nation, between earth and moon, between moon and sun. Out of this idea of separation between atom and atom comes all misery. But the Vedanta says this separation does not exist, it is not real. It is merely apparent, on the surface. In the heart of things there is Unity still. If you go below the surface, you find that Unity between man and man, between races and races, high and low, rich and poor, gods and men, and men and animals. If you go deep enough, all will be seen as only variations of the One, and he who has attained to this conception of Oneness has no more delusion. What can delude him? He knows the reality of everything, the secret of everything. Where is there any more misery for him? What does he desire? He has traced the reality of everything to the Lord, the Centre, the Unity of everything, and that is Eternal Existence, Eternal Knowledge, Eternal Bliss. Neither death nor disease, nor sorrow, nor misery, nor discontent is there. All is Perfect Union and Perfect Bliss. For whom should he mourn then? In the Reality, there is no death, there is no misery; in the Reality, there is no one to mourn for, no one to be sorry for. He has penetrated everything, the Pure One, the Formless, the Bodiless, the Stainless. He the Knower, He the Great Poet, the Self-Existent, He who is giving to everyone what he deserves. They grope in darkness who worship this ignorant world, the world that is produced out of ignorance, thinking of it as Existence, and those who live their whole lives in this world, and never find anything better or higher, are groping in still greater darkness. But he who knows the secret of nature, seeing That which is beyond nature through the help of nature, he crosses death, and through the help of That which is beyond nature, he enjoys Eternal Bliss. "Thou sun, who hast covered the Truth with thy golden disc, do thou remove the veil, so that I may see the Truth that is within thee. I have known the Truth that is within thee, I have known what is the real meaning of thy rays and thy glory and have seen That which shines in thee; the Truth in thee I see, and That which is within thee is within me, and I am That."

❑

8

Realisation

(Delivered in London, 29th October 1896)

I will read to you from one of the Upanishads. It is called the Katha Upanishad. Some of you, perhaps, have read the translation by Sir Edwin Arnold, called the Secret of Death. In our last [i.e. a previous] lecture we saw how the inquiry which started with the origin of the world, and the creation of the universe, failed to obtain a satisfactory answer from without, and how it then turned inwards. This book psychologically takes up that suggestion, questioning into the internal nature of man. It was first asked who created the external world, and how it came into being. Now the question is: What is that in man; which makes him live and move, and what becomes of that when he dies? The first philosophers studied the material substance, and tried to reach the ultimate through that. At the best, they found a personal governor of the universe, a human being immensely magnified, but yet to all intents and purposes a human being. But that could not be the whole of truth; at best, it could be only partial truth. We see this universe as human beings, and our God is our human explanation of the universe.

Suppose a cow were philosophical and had religion it would have a cow universe, and a cow solution of the problem, and it would not be possible that it should see our God. Suppose cats became philosophers, they would see a cat universe and have a cat solution of the problem of the universe, and a cat ruling it. So we see from this that our explanation of the universe is not the whole of the solution. Neither does our conception cover the whole of the universe. It would be a great mistake to accept that tremendously selfish position which man is apt to take. Such a solution of the universal problem as we can get from the outside labours under this difficulty that in the first place the universe we see is our own particular universe, our own view of the Reality. That Reality we cannot see through the senses; we cannot comprehend It. We only know the universe from the point of view of beings with five senses. Suppose we obtain another sense, the whole universe must change for us. Suppose we had a magnetic sense, it is quite possible that we might then find millions and millions of forces in existence which we do not now know, and for which we have no present sense or feeling. Our senses are limited, very limited indeed; and within these limitations exists what we call our universe; and our God is the solution of that universe, but that cannot be the solution of the whole problem. But man cannot stop there. He is a thinking being and wants to find a solution which will comprehensively explain all the universes. He wants to see a world which is at once the world of men, and of gods, and of all possible beings, and to find a solution which will explain all phenomena.

We see, we must first find the universe which includes all universes; we must find something which, by itself, must be the material running through all these various planes of existence, whether we apprehend it through the senses or not. If we could possibly find something which we could know as the common property of the lower as well as of the higher worlds, then our problem would be solved. Even if by the sheer force of logic alone we could understand that there must be one basis of all existence, then our problem might approach to some sort of solution; but this solution certainly cannot be obtained only through the world we see and know, because it is only a partial view of the whole.

Our only hope then lies in penetrating deeper. The early thinkers discovered that the farther they were from; the centre, the more marked were the variations and differentiations; and that the nearer they approached the centre, the nearer they were to unity. The nearer we are to the centre of a circle, the nearer we are to the common ground in which all the radii meet; and the farther we are from the centre, the more divergent is our radial line from the others. The external world is far away from the centre, and so there is no common ground in it where all the phenomena of existence can meet. At best, the external world is but one part of the whole of phenomena. There are other parts, the mental, the moral, and the intellectual – the various planes of existence – and to take up only one, and find a solution of the whole out of that one, is simply impossible. We first, therefore, want to find somewhere a centre from which, as it were, all the other planes of existence start, and standing there we should try to find a solution. That is the proposition. And where is that centre? It is within us. The ancient sages penetrated deeper and deeper until they found that in the innermost core of the human soul is the centre of the whole universe. All the planes gravitate towards that one point. That is the common ground, and standing there alone can we find a common solution. So the question who made this world is not very philosophical, nor does its solution amount to anything.

This the Katha Upanishad speaks in very figurative language. There was, in ancient times, a very rich man, who made a certain sacrifice which required that he should give away everything that he had. Now, this man was not sincere. He wanted to get the fame and glory of having made the sacrifice, but he was only giving things which were of no further use to him – old cows, barren, blind, and lame. He had a boy called Nachiketas. This boy saw that his father was not doing what was right, that he was breaking his vow; but he did not know what to say to him. In India, father and mother are living gods to their children. And so the boy approached the father with the greatest respect and humbly inquired of him, "Father, to whom are you going to give me? For your sacrifice requires that everything shall be given away." The father was very much vexed at this question and replied, "What do you mean, boy? A father giving away his own son?" The boy asked the question a second and a third time, and then the angry father answered, "Thee I give unto Death (Yama)." And the story goes on to say that the boy went to Yama, the god of death. Yama was the first man who died. He went to heaven and became the governor of all the Pitris; all the good people who die, go, and live with him for a long time. He is a very pure and holy person, chaste and good, as his name (Yama) implies.

So the boy went to Yama's world. But even gods are sometimes not at home, and three days this boy had to wait there. After the third day Yama returned. "O learned one," said Yama, "you have been waiting here for three days without food, and you are a guest worthy of respect. Salutation to thee, O Brahmin, and welfare to me! I am very sorry I was not at home. But for that I will make amends. Ask three boons, one for each day." And the boy asked, "My first boon is that my father's anger against me may pass away; that he will be kind to me and recognise me when you allow me to depart." Yama granted this fully. The next boon was that he wanted to know about a certain sacrifice which took people to heaven. Now we have seen that the oldest idea which we got in the Samhitâ portion of the Vedas was only about heaven where they had bright bodies and lived with the fathers. Gradually other ideas came, but they were not satisfying; there was still need for something higher. Living in heaven would not be very different from life in this world. At best, it would only be a very healthy rich man's life, with plenty of sense-enjoyments and a sound body which knows no disease. It would be this material world, only a little more refined; and we have seen the difficulty that the external material world can never solve the problem. So no heaven can solve the problem. If this world cannot solve the problem, no multiplication of this world can do so, because we must always remember that matter is only an infinitesimal part of the phenomena of nature. The vast part of phenomena which we actually see is not matter. For instance, in every moment of our life what a great part is played by thought and feeling, compared with the material phenomena outside! How vast is this internal world with its tremendous activity! The sense-phenomena are very small compared with it. The heaven solution commits this mistake; it insists that the whole of phenomena is only in touch, taste, sight, etc. So this idea of heaven did not give full satisfaction to all. Yet

Nachiketas asks, as the second boon, about some sacrifice through which people might attain to this heaven. There was an idea in the Vedas that these sacrifices pleased the gods and took human beings to heaven.

In studying all religions you will notice the fact that whatever is old becomes holy. For instance, our forefathers in India used to write on birch bark, but in time they learnt how to make paper. Yet the birch bark is still looked upon as very holy. When the utensils in which they used to cook in ancient times were improved upon, the old ones became holy; and nowhere is this idea more kept up than in India. Old methods, which must be nine or ten thousand years old, as of rubbing two sticks together to make fire, are still followed. At the time of sacrifice no other method will do. So with the other branch of the Asiatic Aryans. Their modern descendants still like to obtain fire from lightning, showing that they used to get fire in this way. Even when they learnt other customs, they kept up the old ones, which then became holy. So with the Hebrews. They used to write on parchment. They now write on paper, but parchment is very holy. So with all nations. Every rite which you now consider holy was simply an old custom, and the Vedic sacrifice were of this nature. In course of time, as they found better methods of life, their ideas were much improved; still these old forms remained, and from time to time they were practiced and received a holy significance.

Then, a body of men made it their business to carry on these sacrifices. These were the priests, who speculated on the sacrifices, and the sacrifices became everything to them. The gods came to enjoy the fragrance of the sacrifices, and it was considered that everything in this world could be got by the power of sacrifices. If certain oblations were made, certain hymns chanted, certain peculiar forms of altars made, the gods would grant everything. So Nachiketas asks by what form of sacrifice can a man go to heaven. The second boon was also readily granted by Yama who promised that this sacrifice should henceforth be named after Nachiketas.

Then the third boon comes, and with that the Upanishad proper begins. The boy said, "There is this difficulty: when a man dies some say he is, others that he is not. Instructed by you I desire to understand this." But Yama was frightened. He had been very glad to grant the other two boons. Now he said, "The gods in ancient times were puzzled on this point. This subtle law is not easy to understand. Choose some other boon, O Nachiketas, do not press me on this point, release me."

The boy was determined, and said, "What you have said is true, O Death, that even the gods had doubts on this point, and it is no easy matter to understand. But I cannot obtain another exponent like you and there is no other boon equal to this."

Death said, "Ask for sons and grandsons who will live one hundred years, many cattle, elephants, gold, and horses. Ask for empire on this earth and live as many ears as you like. Or choose any other boon which you think equal to these – wealth and long life. Or be thou a king, O Nachiketas, on the wide earth. I will make thee the enjoyer of all desires. Ask for all those desires which are difficult to obtain in the world. These heavenly maidens with chariots and music, which are not to be obtained by man, are yours. Let them serve you. O Nachiketas, but do not question me as to what comes after death."

Nachiketas said, "These are merely things of a day, O Death, they wear away the energy of all the sense-organs. Even the longest life is very short. These horses and chariots, dances and songs, may remain with Thee. Man cannot be satisfied by wealth. Can we retain wealth when we behold Thee? We shall live only so long as Thou desires". Only the boon which I have asked is chosen by me."

Yama was pleased with this answer and said, "Perfection is one thing and enjoyment another; these two having different ends, engage men differently. He who chooses perfection becomes pure. He who chooses enjoyment misses his true end. Both perfection and enjoyment present themselves to man; the wise man having examined both distinguishes one from the other. He chooses perfection as being superior to enjoyment, but the foolish man chooses enjoyment for the pleasure of his body. O Nachiketas, having thought upon the things which are only apparently desirable, thou hast wisely abandoned them." Death then proceeded to teach Nachiketas.

We now get a very developed idea of renunciation and Vedic morality, that until one has conquered the desires for enjoyment the truth will not shine in him. So long as these vain desires of our senses are clamouring and as it were dragging us outwards every moment, making us slaves to everything outside – to a little colour, a little taste, a little touch – notwithstanding all our pretensions, how can the truth express itself in our hearts?

Yama said, "That which is beyond never rises before the mind of a thoughtless child deluded by the folly of riches. 'This world exists, the other does not,' thinking thus they come again and again under my power. To understand this truth is very difficult. Many, even hearing it continually, do not understand it, for the speaker must be wonderful, so must be the hearer. The teacher must be wonderful, so must be the taught. Neither is the mind to be disturbed By vain arguments, for it is no more a question of argument, it is a question of fact." We have always heard that every religion insists on our having faith. We have been taught to believe blindly. Well, this idea of blind faith is objectionable, no doubt, but analysing it, we find that behind it is a very great truth. What it really means is what we read now. The mind is not to be ruffled by vain arguments, because argument will not help us to know God. It is a question of fact, and not of argument. All argument and reasoning must be based upon certain perceptions. Without these, there cannot be any argument. Reasoning is the method of comparison between certain facts which we have already perceived. If these perceived facts are not there already, there cannot be any reasoning. If this is true of external phenomena, why should it not be so of the internal? The chemist takes certain chemicals and certain results are produced. This is a fact; you see it, sense it, and make that the basis on which to build all your chemical arguments. So with the physicists, so with all other sciences. All knowledge must stand on perception of certain facts, and upon that we have to build our reasoning. But, curiously enough the vast majority of mankind think, especially at the present time, that no such perception is possible in religion, that religion can only be apprehended by vain arguments. Therefore we are told not to disturb the mind by vain arguments. Religion is a question of fact, not of talk. We have to analyse our own souls and to find what is there. We have to understand it and to realise what is understood. That is religion. No amount of talk will make religion. So the question whether there is a God or not can never be proved by argument, for the arguments are as much on one side as on the other. But if there is a God, He is in our own hearts. Have you ever seen Him? The question as to whether this world exists or not has not yet been decided, and the debate between the idealists and the realists is endless. Yet we know that the world exists, that it goes on. We only change the meaning of words. So, with all the questions of life, we must come to facts. There are certain religious facts which, as in external science, have to be perceived, and upon them religion will be built. Of course, the extreme claim that you must believe every dogma of a religion is degrading to the human mind. The man who asks you to believe everything, degrades himself, and, if you believe, degrades you too. The sages of the world have only the right to tell us that they have analysed their minds and have found these facts, and if we do the same we shall also believe, and not before. That is all that there is in religion. But you must always remember this, that as a matter of fact 99.9 per cent of those who attack religion have never analysed their minds, have never struggled to get at the facts. So their arguments do not have any weight against religion, any more than the words of a blind man who cries out, "You are all fools who believe in the sun," would affect us.

This is one great idea to learn and to hold on to, this idea of realisation. This turmoil and fight and difference in religions will cease only when we understand that religion is not in books and temples. It is an actual perception. Only the man who has actually perceived God and soul has religion. There is no real difference between the highest ecclesiastical giant who can talk by the volume, and the lowest, most ignorant materialist. We are all atheists; let us confess it. Mere intellectual assent does not make us religious. Take a Christian, or a Mohammedan, or a follower of any other religion in the world. Any man who truly realised the truth of the Sermon on the Mount would be perfect, and become a god immediately. Yet it is said that there are many millions of Christians in the world. What is meant is that mankind may at some time try to realise that Sermon. Not one in twenty millions is a real Christian.

So, in India, there are said to be three hundred millions of Vedantins. But if there were one in a thousand who had actually realised religion, this world would soon be greatly changed. We are all atheists, and yet we try to fight the man who admits it. We are all in the dark; religion is to us a mere intellectual assent, a mere talk, a mere nothing. We often consider a man religious who can talk well. But this is not religion. "Wonderful methods of joining words, rhetorical powers, and explaining texts of the books in various ways – these are only for the enjoyment of the learned, and not religion." Religion comes when that actual realisation in our own souls begins. That will be the dawn of religion; and then alone we shall be moral. Now we are not much more moral than the animals. We are only held down by the whips of society. If society said today, "I will not punish you if you steal", we should just make a rush for each other's property. It is the policeman that makes us moral. It is social opinion that makes us moral, and really we are little better than animals. We understand how much this is so in the secret of our own hearts. So let us not be hypocrites. Let us confess that we are not religious and have no right to look down on others. We are all brothers and we shall be truly moral when we have realised religion.

If you have seen a certain country, and a man forces you to say that you have not seen it, still in your heart of hearts you know you have. So, when you see religion and God in a more intense sense than you see this external world, nothing will be able to shake your belief. Then you have real faith. That is what is meant by the words in your Gospel, "He who has faith even as a grain of mustard seed." Then you will know the Truth because you have become the Truth.

This is the watchword of the Vedanta — realise religion, no talking will do. But it is done with great difficulty. He has hidden Himself inside the atom, this Ancient One who resides in the inmost recess of every human heart. The sages realised Him through the power of introspection, and got beyond both joy and misery, beyond what we call virtue and vice, beyond good and bad deeds, beyond being and non-being; he who has seen Him has seen the Reality. But what then about heaven? It was the idea of happiness minus unhappiness. That is to say, what we want is the joys of this life minus its sorrows. That is a very good idea, no doubt; it comes naturally; but it is a mistake throughout, because there is no such thing as absolute good, nor any such thing as absolute evil.

You have all heard of that rich man in Rome who learnt one day that he had only about a million pounds of his property left; he said, "What shall I do tomorrow?" and forthwith committed suicide. A million pounds was poverty to him. What is joy, and what is sorrow? It is a vanishing quantity, continually vanishing. When I was a child I thought if I could be a cabman, it would be the very acme of happiness for me to drive about. I do not think so now. To what joy will you cling? This is the one point we must all try to understand, and it is one of the last superstitions to leave us. Everyone's idea of pleasure is different. I have seen a man who is not happy unless he swallows a lump of opium every day. He may dream of a heaven where the land is made of opium. That would be a very bad heaven for me. Again and again in Arabian poetry we read of heaven with beautiful gardens, through which rivers run. I lived much of my life in a country where there is too much water; many villages are flooded and thousands of lives are sacrificed every year. So, my heaven would not have gardens through which rivers flow; I would have a land where very little rain falls. Our pleasures are always changing. If a young man dreams of heaven, he dreams of a heaven where he will have a beautiful wife. When that same man becomes old he does not want a wife. It is our necessities which make our heaven, and the heaven changes with the change of our necessities. If we had a heaven like that desired by those to whom sense-enjoyment is the very end of existence, then we would not progress. That would be the most terrible curse we could pronounce on the soul. Is this all we can come to? A little weeping and dancing, and then to die like a dog! What a curse you pronounce on the head of humanity when you long for these things! That is what you do when you cry after the joys of this world, for you do not know what true joy is. What philosophy insists on is not to give up joys, but to know what joy really is. The Norwegian heaven is a tremendous fighting place where they all sit before Odin; they have a wild boar hunt, and then they go to war and slash each other to pieces. But in some way or other, after a few hours of such fighting, the wounds are all healed up, and they go into a hall where the boar has been roasted, and have a carousal. And then the wild boar takes form again, ready to be hunted the next day. That is much the same thing as our heaven, not a whit worse, only our ideas may be a little more refined. We want to hunt wild boars, and get to a place where all enjoyments will continue, just as the Norwegian imagines that the wild boar is hunted and eaten every day, and recovers the next day.

Now, philosophy insists that there is a joy which is absolute, which never changes. That joy cannot be the joys and pleasures we have in this life, and yet Vedanta shows that everything that is joyful in this life is but a particle of that real joy, because that is the only joy there is. Every moment really we are enjoying the absolute bliss, though covered up, misunderstood, and caricatured. Wherever there is any blessing, blissfulness, or joy, even the joy of the thief in stealing, it is that absolute bliss coming out, only it has become obscured, muddled up, as it were, with all sorts of extraneous conditions, and misunderstood. But to understand that, we have to go through the negation, and then the positive side will begin. We have to give up ignorance and all that is false, and then truth will begin to reveal itself to us. When we have grasped the truth, things which we gave up at first will take new shape and form, will appear to us in a new light, and become deified. They will have become sublimated, and then we shall understand them in their true light. But to understand them, we have first to get a glimpse of truth; we must give them up at first, and then we get them back again, deified. We have to give up all our miseries and sorrows, all our little joys.

"That which all the Vedas declare, which is proclaimed by all penances, seeking which men lead lives of continence, I will tell you in one word — it is 'Om'." You will find this word "Om" praised very much in the Vedas, and it is held to be very sacred.

Now Yama answers the question: "What becomes of a man when the body dies ?" "This Wise One never dies, is never born, It arises from nothing, and nothing arises from It. Unborn, Eternal, Everlasting, this Ancient One can never be destroyed with the destruction of the body. If the slayer thinks he can slay, or if the slain thinks he is slain, they both do not know the truth, for the Self neither slays nor is slain." A most tremendous position. I should like to draw your attention to the adjective in the first line, which is "wise". As we proceed we shall find that the ideal of the Vedanta is that all wisdom and all purity are in the soul already, dimly expressed or better expressed — that is all the difference. The difference between man and man, and all things in the whole creation, is not in kind but only in degree. The background, the reality, of everyone is that same Eternal, Ever Blessed, Ever Pure, and Ever Perfect One. It is the Atman, the Soul, in the saint and the sinner, in the happy and the miserable, in the beautiful and the ugly, in men and in animals; it is the same throughout. It is the shining One. The difference is caused by the power of expression. In some It is expressed more, in others less, but this difference of expression has no effect upon the Atman. If in their dress one man shows more of his body than another, it does not make any difference in their bodies; the difference is in their dress. We had better remember here that throughout the Vedanta philosophy, there is no such thing as good and bad, they are not two different things; the same thing is good or bad, and the difference is only in degree. The very thing I call pleasurable today, tomorrow under better circumstances I may call pain. The fire that warms us can also consume us; it is not the fault of the fire. Thus, the Soul being pure and perfect, the man who does evil is giving the lie unto himself, he does not know the nature of himself. Even in the murderer the pure Soul is there; It dies not. It was his mistake; he could not manifest It; he had covered It up. Nor in the man who thinks that he is killed is the Soul killed; It is eternal. It can never be killed, never destroyed. "Infinitely smaller than the smallest, infinitely larger than the largest, this Lord of all is present in the depths of every human heart. The sinless, bereft of all misery, see Him through the mercy of the Lord; the Bodiless, yet dwelling in the body; the Spaceless, yet seeming to occupy space; Infinite, Omnipresent: knowing such to be the Soul, the sages never are miserable."

"This Atman is not to be realised by the power of speech, nor by a vast intellect, nor by the study of their Vedas." This is a very bold utterance. As I told you before, the sages were very bold thinkers, and never stopped at anything. You will remember that in India these Vedas are regarded in a much higher light than even the Christians regard their Bible. Your idea of revelation is that a man was inspired by God; but in India the idea is that things exist because they are in the Vedas. In and through the Vedas the whole creation has come. All that is called knowledge is in the Vedas. Every word is sacred and eternal, eternal as the soul, without beginning and without end. The whole of the Creator's mind is in this book, as it were. That is the light in which the Vedas are held. Why is this thing moral? Because the Vedas say so. Why is that thing immoral? Because the Vedas say so. In spite of that, look at the boldness of these sages whom proclaimed that the truth is not to be found by much study of the Vedas. "With whom the Lord is pleased, to that man He expresses Himself." But then, the objection may be advanced that this is something like partisanship. But at Yama explains, "Those who are evil-doers, whose minds area not peaceful, can never see the Light. It is to those who are true in heart, pure in deed, whose senses are controlled, that this Self manifests Itself."

Here is a beautiful figure. Picture the Self to be then rider and this body the chariot, the intellect to be the charioteer, mind the reins, and the senses the horses. He whose horses are well broken, and whose reins are strong and kept well in the hands of the charioteer (the intellect) reaches the goal which is the state of Him, the Omnipresent. But the man whose horses (the senses) are not controlled, nor the reins (the mind) well managed, goes to destruction. This Atman in all beings does not manifest Himself to the eyes or the senses, but those whose minds have become purified and refined realise Him. Beyond all sound, all sight, beyond form, absolute, beyond all taste and touch, infinite, without beginning and without end, even beyond nature, the Unchangeable; he who realises Him, frees himself from the jaws of death. But it is very difficult. It is, as it were, walking on the edge of a razor; the way is long and perilous, but struggle on, do not despair. Awake, arise, and stop not till the goal is reached.

The one central idea throughout all the Upanishads is that of realisation. A great many questions will arise from time to time, and especially to the modern man. There will be the question of utility, there will be various other questions, but in all we shall find that we are prompted by our past associations. It is association of ideas that has such a tremendous power over our minds. To those who from childhood have always heard of a Personal God and the personality of the mind, these ideas will of course appear very stern and harsh, but if they listen to them and think over them, they will become part of their lives and will no longer frighten them. The great question that generally arises is the utility of philosophy. To that there can be only one answer: if on the utilitarian ground it is good for men to seek for pleasure, why should not those whose pleasure is in religious speculation seek for that? Because sense-enjoyments please many, they seek for them, but there may be others whom they do not please, who want higher enjoyment. The dog's pleasure is only in eating and drinking. The dog cannot understand the pleasure of the scientist who gives up everything, and, perhaps, dwells on the top of a mountain to observe the position of certain stars. The dogs may smile at him and think he is a madman. Perhaps this poor scientist never had money enough to marry even, and lives very simply. May be, the dog laughs at him. But the scientist says, "My dear dog, your pleasure is only in the senses which you enjoy, and you know nothing beyond; but for me this is the most enjoyable life, and if you have the right to seek your pleasure in your own way, so have I in mine." The mistake is that we want to tie the whole world down to our own plane of thought and to make our mind the measure of the whole universe. To you, the old sense-things are, perhaps, the greatest pleasure, but it is not necessary that my pleasure should be the same, and when you insist upon that, I differ from you. That is the difference between the worldly utilitarian and the religious man. The first man says, "See how happy I am. I get money, but do not bother my head about religion. It is too unsearchable, and I am happy without it." So far, so good; good for all utilitarians. But this world is terrible. If a man gets happiness in any way excepting by injuring his fellow-beings, godspeed him; but when this man comes to me and says, "You too must do these things, you will be a fool if you do not," I say, "You are wrong, because the very things, which are pleasurable to you, have not the slightest attraction for me. If I had to go after a few handfuls of gold, my life would not be worth living! I should die." That is the answer the religious man would make. The fact is that religion is possible only for those who have finished with these lower things. We must have our own experiences, must have our full run. It is only when we have finished this run that the other world opens.

The enjoyments of the senses sometimes assume another phase which is dangerous and tempting. You will always hear the idea — in very old times, in every religion — that a time will come when all the miseries of life wills cease, and only its joys and pleasures will remain, and this earth will become a heaven. That I do not believe. This earth will always remain this same world. It is a most terrible thing to say, yet I do not see my way out of it. The misery in the world is like chronic rheumatism in the body; drive it from one part and it goes to another, drive it from there and you will feel it somewhere else. Whatever you do, it is still there. In olden times people lived in forests, and ate each other; in modern times they do not eat each other's flesh, but they cheat one another. Whole countries and cities are ruined by cheating. That does not show much progress. I do not see that what you call progress in the world is other than the multiplication of desires. If one thing is obvious to me it is this that desires bring all misery; it is the state of the beggar, who is always begging for something, and unable to see anything without the wish to possess it, is always longing, longing for more. If the power to satisfy our desires is increased in arithmetical progression, the power of desire is increased in geometrical progression. The sum total of happiness and misery in this world is at least the same throughout. If a wave rises in the ocean it makes a hollow somewhere. If happiness comes to one man, unhappiness comes to another or, perhaps, to some animal. Men are increasing in numbers and some animals are decreasing; we are killing them off, and taking their land ; we are taking all means of sustenance from them. How can we say, then, that happiness is increasing? The strong race eats up the weaker, but do you think that the strong race will be very happy? No; they will begin to kill each other. I do not see on practical grounds how this world can become a heaven. Facts are against it. On theoretical grounds also, I see it cannot be.

Perfection is always infinite. We are this infinite already, and we are trying to manifest that infinity. You and I, and all beings, are trying to manifest it. So far it is all right. But from this fact some German philosophers have started a peculiar theory — that this manifestation will become higher and higher until we attain perfect manifestation, until we have become perfect beings. What is meant by perfect manifestation? Perfection means infinity, and manifestation means limit, and so it means that we shall become unlimited limiteds, which is self-contradictory. Such a theory may please children; but it is poisoning their minds with lies, and is very bad for religion. But we know that this world is a degradation, that man is a degradation of God, and that Adam fell. There is no religion today that does not teach that man is a degradation. We have been degraded down to the animal, and are now going up, to emerge out of this bondage. But we shall never be able entirely to manifest the Infinite here. We shall struggle hard, but there will come a time when we shall find that it is impossible to be perfect here, while we are bound by the senses. And then the march back to our original state of Infinity will be sounded.

This is renunciation. We shall have to get out of the difficulty by reversing the process by which we got in, and then morality and charity will begin. What is the watchword of all ethical codes? "Not I, but thou", and this "I" is the outcome of the Infinite behind, trying to manifest Itself on the outside world. This little "I" is the result, and it will have to go back and join the Infinite, its own nature. Every time you say, "Not I, my brother, but thou", you are trying to go back, and every time you say "I, and not thou", you take the false step of trying to manifest the Infinite through the sense-world. That brings struggles and evils into the world, but after a time renunciation must come, eternal renunciation. The little "I" is dead and gone. Why care so much for this little life? All these vain desires of living and enjoying this life, here or in some other place, bring death.

If we are developed from animals, the animals also may be degraded men. How do you know it is not so? You have seen that the proof of evolution is simply this: you find a series of bodies from the lowest to the highest rising in a gradually ascending scale. But from that how can you insist that it is always from the lower upwards, and never from the higher downwards? The argument applies both ways, and if anything is true, I believe it is that the series is repeating itself in going up and down. How can you have evolution without involution? Our struggle for the higher life shows that we have been degraded from a high state. It must be so, only it may vary as to details. I always cling to the idea set forth with one voice by Christ, Buddha, and the Vedanta, that we must all come to perfection in time, but only by giving up this imperfection. This world is nothing. It is at best only a hideous caricature, a shadow of the Reality. We must go to the Reality. Renunciation will take us to It. Renunciation is the very basis of our true life; every moment of goodness and real life that we enjoy is when we do not think of ourselves. This little separate self must die. Then we shall find that we are in the Real, and that Reality is God, and He is our own true nature, and He is always in us and with us. Let us live in Him and stand in Him. It is the only joyful state of existence. Life on the plane of the Spirit is the only life, and let us all try to attain to this realisation.

❑

9

Unity in Diversity

(Delivered in London, 3rd November 1896)

"The Self-existent One projected the senses outwards and, therefore, a man looks outward, not within himself. A certain wise one, desiring immortality, with inverted senses, perceived the Self within." As I have already said, the first inquiry that we find in the Vedas was concerning outward things, and then a new idea came that the reality of things is not to be found in the external world; not by looking outwards, but by turning the eyes, as it is literally expressed, inwards. And the word used for the Soul is very significant: it is He who has gone inward, the innermost reality of our being, the heart centre, the core, from which, as it were, everything comes out; the central sun of which the mind, the body, the sense-organs, and everything else we have are but rays going outwards. "Men of childish intellect, ignorant persons, run after desires which are external, and enter the trap of far-reaching death, but the wise, understanding immortality, never seek for the Eternal in this life of finite things." The same idea is here made clear that in this external world, which is full of finite things, it is impossible to see and find the Infinite. The Infinite must be sought in that alone which is infinite, and the only thing infinite about us is that which is within us, our own soul. Neither the body, nor the mind, not even our thoughts, nor the world we see around us, are infinite. The Seer, He to whom they all belong, the Soul of man, He who is awake in the internal man, alone is infinite, and to seek for the Infinite Cause of this whole universe we must go there. In the

Infinite Soul alone we can find it. "What is here is there too, and what is there is here also. He who sees the manifold goes from death to death." We have seen how at first there was the desire to go to heaven. When these ancient Aryans became dissatisfied with the world around them, they naturally thought that after death they would go to some place where there would be all happiness without any misery; these places they multiplied and called Svargas – the word may be translated as heavens – where there would be joy for ever, the body would become perfect, and also the mind, and there they would live with their forefathers. But as soon as philosophy came, men found that this was impossible and absurd. The very idea of an infinite in place would be a contradiction in terms, as a place must begin and continue in time. Therefore they had to give up that idea. They found out that the gods who lived in these heavens had once been human beings on earth, who through their good works had become gods, and the godhoods, as they call them, were different states, different positions; none of the gods spoken of in the Vedas are permanent individuals.

For instance, Indra and Varuna are not the names of certain persons, but the names of positions as governors and so on. The Indra who had lived before is not the same person as the Indra of the present day; he has passed away, and another man from earth has filled his place. So with all the other gods These are certain positions, which are filled successively by human souls who have raised themselves to the condition of gods, and yet even they die. In the old Rig-Veda we find the word "immortality" used with regard to these gods, but later on it is dropped entirely, for they found that immortality which is beyond time and space cannot be spoken of with regard to any physical form, however subtle it may be. However fine it may be, it must have a beginning in time and space, for the necessary factors that enter into the make-up of form are in space. Try to think of a form without space: it is impossible. Space is one of the materials, as it were, which make up the form, and this is continually changing Space and time are in Maya, and this idea is expressed in the line – "What is hole, that is there too." If there are these gods, they must be bound by the same laws that apply here, and all laws involve destruction and renewal again and again. These laws are moulding matter into different forms, and crushing them out again. Everything born must die; and so, if there are heavens, the same laws must hold good there.

In this world we find that all happiness is followed by misery as its shadow. Life has its shadow, death. They must go together, because they are not contradictory, not two separate existences, but different manifestations of the same unit, life and death, sorrow and happiness, good and evil. The dualistic conception that good and evil are two separate entities, and that they are both going on eternally is absurd on the face of it. They are the diverse manifestations of one and the same fact, one time appearing as bad, and at another time as good. The difference does not exist in kind, but only in degree. They differ from each other in degree of intensity. We find as a fact that the same nerve systems carry good and bad sensations alike, and when the nerves are injured, neither sensation comes to us. If a certain nerve is paralysed, we do not get the pleasurable feelings that used to come along that wires and at the same time we do not get the painful feelings either. They are never two, but the same. Again. the same thing produces pleasure and pain at different times of life. The same phenomenon will produce pleasure in one, and pain in another. The eating of meat produces pleasure to a man, but pain to the animal which is eaten. There has never been anything which gives pleasure to all alike. Some are pleased, others displeased. So on it will go. Therefore, this duality of existence is denied. And what follows? I told you in my last lecture that we can never have ultimately everything good on this earth and nothing bad. It may have disappointed and frightened some of you, but I cannot help it, and I am open to conviction when I am shown to the contrary; but until that can be proved to me, and I can find that it is true, cannot say so.

The general argument against my statement, and apparently a very convincing one, is this that in the course of evolution, all that is evil in what we see around us is gradually being eliminated, and the result is that if this elimination continues for millions of years, a time will come when all the evil will have been extirpated, and the good alone will remain. This is apparently a very sound argument. Would to God it were true! But there is a fallacy in it, and it is this that it takes for granted that both good and evil are things that are eternally fixed. It takes for granted that there is a definite mass of evil, which may be represented by a hundred, and likewise of good, and that this mass of evil is being diminished every day, leaving only the good. But is it so? The history of the world shows that evil is a continuously increasing quantity, as well as good. Take the lowest man; he lives in the forest. His sense of enjoyment is very small, and so also is his power to suffer. His misery is entirely on the sense-plane. If he does not get plenty of food, he is miserable; but give him plenty of food and freedom to rove and to hunt, and he is perfectly happy. His happiness consists only in the senses, and so does his misery also. But if that man increases in knowledge, his happiness will increase, the intellect will open to him, and his sense-enjoyment will evolve into intellectual enjoyment. He will feel pleasure in reading a beautiful poem, and a mathematical problem will be of absorbing interest to him. But, with these, the inner nerves will become more and more susceptible to miseries of mental pain, of which the savage does not think. Take a very simple illustration. In Tibet there is no marriage, and there is no jealousy, yet we know that marriage is a much higher state. The Tibetans have not known the wonderful enjoyment, the blessing of chastity, the happiness of having a chaste, virtuous wife, or a chaste, virtuous husband. These people cannot feel that. And similarly they do not feel the intense jealousy of the chaste wife or husband, or the misery caused by unfaithfulness on either side, with all the heart-burnings and sorrows which believers in chastity experience. On one side, the latter gain happiness, but on the other, they suffer misery too.

Take your country which is the richest in the world, and which is more luxurious than any other, and see how intense is the misery, how many more lunatics you have, compared with other races, only because the desires are so keen. A man must keep up a high standard of living, and the amount of money he spends in one year would be a fortune to a man in India. You cannot preach to him of simple living because society demands so much of him. The wheel of society is rolling on; it stops not for the widow's tears or the orphans' wails. This is the state of things everywhere. Your sense of enjoyment is developed, your society is very much more beautiful than some others. You have so many more things to enjoy. But those who have fewer have much less misery. You can argue thus throughout, the higher the ideal you have in the brain, the greater is your enjoyment, and the more profound your misery. One is like the shadow of the other. That the evils are being eliminated may be true, but if so, the good also must be dying out. But are not evils multiplying fast, and good diminishing, if I may so put it? If good increases in arithmetical progression, evil increase in geometrical progression. And this is Maya. This is neither optimism nor pessimism. Vedanta does not take he position that this world is only a miserable one. That would be untrue. At the same time, it is a mistake to say that this world is full of happiness and blessings. So it is useless to tell children that this world is all good, all flowers, all milk and honey. That is what we have all dreamt. At the same time it is erroneous to think, because one man has suffered more than another, that all is evil. It is this duality, this play of good and evil that makes our world of experiences. At the same time the Vedanta says, "Do not think that good and evil are two, are two separate essences, for they are one and the same thing, appearing in different degrees and in different guises and producing differences of feeling in the same mind." So, the first thought of the Vedanta is the finding of unity in the external; the One Existence manifesting Itself, however different It may appear in manifestation. Think of the old crude theory of the Persians — two gods creating this world, the good god doing everything that is good, and the bad one, everything bad. On the very face of it, you see the absurdity, for if it be carried out, every law of nature must have two parts, one of which is manipulated by one god, and then he goes away and the other god manipulates the other part. There the difficulty comes that both are working in the same world, and these two gods keep themselves in harmony by injuring one portion and doing good to another. This is a crude case, of course, the crudest way of expressing the duality of existence. But, take the more advanced, the more abstract theory that this world is partly good and partly bad. This also is absurd, arguing from the same standpoint. It is the law of unity that gives us our food, and it is the same law that kills many through accidents or misadventure.

We find, then, that this world is neither optimistic nor pessimistic; it is a mixture of both, and as we go on we shall find that the whole blame is taken away from nature and put upon our own shoulders. At the same time the Vedanta shows the way out, but not by denial of evil, because it analyses boldly the fact as it is and does not seek to conceal anything. It is not hopeless; it is not agnostic. It finds out a remedy, but it wants to place that remedy on adamantine foundations: not by shutting the child's mouth and blinding its eyes with something which is untrue, and which the child will find out in a few days. I remember when I was young, a young man's father died and left him poorly off, with a large family to support, and he found that his father's friends were unwilling to help him. He had a conversation with a clergyman who offered this consolation, "Oh, it is all good, all is sent for our good." That is the old method of trying to put a piece of gold leaf on an old sore. It is a confession of weakness, of absurdity. The young man went away, and six months afterwards a son was born to the clergyman, and he gave a thanksgiving party to which the young man was invited. The clergyman prayed, "Thank God for His mercies." And the young man stood up and said, "Stop, this is all misery." The clergyman asked, "Why?" "Because when my father died you said it was good, though apparently evil; so now, this is apparently good, but really evil." Is this the way to cure the misery of the world? Be good and have mercy on those who suffer. Do not try to patch it up, nothing will cure this world; go beyond it.

This is a world of good and evil. Wherever there is good, evil follows, but beyond and behind all these manifestations, all these contradictions, the Vedanta finds out that Unity. It says, "Give up what is evil and give up what is good." What remains then? Behind good and evil stands something which is yours, the real you, beyond every evil, and beyond every good too, and it is that which is manifesting itself as good and bad. Know that first, and then and then alone you will be a true optimist, and not before; for then you will be able to control everything. Control these manifestations and you will be at liberty to manifest the real "you". First be master of yourself, stand up and be free, go beyond the pale of these laws, for these laws do not absolutely govern you, they are only part of your being. First find out that you are not the slave of nature, never were and never will be; that this nature, infinite as you may think it, is only finite, a drop in the ocean, and your Soul is the ocean; you are beyond the stars, the sun, and the moon. They are like mere bubbles compared with your infinite being. Know that, and you will control both good and evil. Then alone the whole vision will change and you will stand up and say, "How beautiful is good and how wonderful is evil!"

That is what the Vedanta teaches. It does not propose any slipshod remedy by covering wounds with gold leaf and the more the wound festers, putting on more gold leaf. This life is a hard fact; work your way through it boldly, though it may be adamantine; no matter, the soul is stronger. It lays no responsibility on little gods; for you are the makers of your own fortunes. You make yourselves suffer, you make good and evil, and it is you who put your hands before your eyes and say it is dark. Take your hands away and see the light; you are effulgent, you are perfect already, from the very beginning. We now understand the verse: "He goes from death to death who sees the many here." See that One and be free.

How are we to see it? This mind, so deluded, so weak, so easily led, even this mind can be strong and may catch a glimpse of that knowledge, that Oneness, which saves us from dying again and again. As rain falling upon a mountain flows in various streams down the sides of the mountain, so all the energies which you see here are from that one Unit. It has become manifold falling upon Maya. Do not run after the manifold; go towards the One. "He is in all that moves; He is in all that is pure; He fills the universe; He is in the sacrifice; He is the guest in the house; He is in man, in water, in animals, in truth; He is the Great One. As fire coming into this world is manifesting itself in various forms, even so, that one Soul of the universe is manifesting Himself in all these various forms. As air coming into this universe manifests itself in various forms, even so, the One Soul of all souls, of all beings, is manifesting Himself in all forms." This is true for you when you have understood this Unity, and not before Then is all optimism, because He is seen everywhere. The question is that if all this be true that that Pure One – the Self, the Infinite – has entered all this, how is it that He suffers, how is it that He becomes miserable, impure? He does not, says the Upanishad. "As the sun is the cause of the eyesight of every being, yet is not made defective by the defect in any eye, even so the Self of all is not affected by the miseries of the body, or by any misery that is around you." I may have some disease and see everything yellow, but the sun is not affected by it. "He is the One, the Creator of all, the Ruler of all, the Internal Soul of every being – He who makes His Oneness manifold. Thus sages who realise Him as the Soul of their souls, unto them belongs eternal peace; unto none else, unto none else. He who in this world of evanescence finds Him who never changes, he who in this universe of death finds that One Life, he who in this manifold finds that Oneness, and all those who realise Him as the Soul of their souls, to them belongs eternal peace; unto none else, unto none else. Where to find Him in the external world, where to find Him in the suns, and moons, and stars? There the sun cannot illumine, nor the moon, nor the stars, the flash of lightning cannot illumine the place; what to speak of this mortal fire? He shining, everything else shines. It is His light that they have borrowed, and He is shining through them." Here is another beautiful simile. Those of you who have been in India and have seen how the banyan tree comes from one root and spreads itself far around, will understand this. He is that banyan tree; He is the root of all and has branched out until He has become this universe, and however far He extends, every one of these trunks and branches is connected.

Various heavens are spoken of in the Brâhmana portions of the Vedas, but the philosophical teaching of the Upanishads gives up the idea of going to heaven. Happiness is not in this heaven or in that heaven, it is in the soul; places do not signify anything. Here is another passage which shows the different states of realisation "In the heaven of the forefathers, as a man sees things in a dream, so the Real Truth is seen." As in dreams we see things hazy and not so distinct, so we see the Reality there. There is another heaven called the Gandharva, in which it is still less clear; as a man sees his own reflection in the water, so is the Reality seen there. The highest heaven, of which the Hindus conceive is called the Brahmaloka; and in this, the Truth is seen much more clearly, like light and shade, but not yet quite distinctly. But as a man sees his own face in a mirror, perfect, distinct, and clear, so is the Truth shining in the soul of man. The highest heaven, therefore, is in our own souls; the greatest temple of worship is the human soul, greater than all heavens, says the Vedanta; for in no heaven anywhere, can we understand the reality as distinctly and clearly as in this life, in our own soul. Changing places does not help one much. I thought while I was in India that the cave would give me clearer vision. I found it was not so. Then I thought the forest would do so, then, Varanasi. But the same difficulty existed everywhere, because we make our own worlds. If I am evil, the whole world is evil to me. That is what the Upanishad says. And the same thing applies to all worlds. If I die and go to heaven, I should find the same, for until I am pure it is no use going to caves, or forests, or to Varanasi, or to heaven, and if I have polished my mirror, it does not matter where I live, I get the Reality just as It is. So it is useless, running hither and thither, and spending energy in vain, which should be spent only in polishing the mirror. The same idea is expressed again: "None sees Him, none sees His form with the eyes. It is in the mind, in the pure mind, that He is seen, and this immortality is gained."

Those who were at the summer lectures on Râja-Yoga will be interested to know that what was taught then was a different kind of Yoga. The Yoga which we are now considering consists chiefly in controlling the senses. When the senses are held as slaves by the human soul, when they can no longer disturb the mind, then the Yogi has reached the goal. "When all vain desires of the heart have been given up, then this very mortal becomes immortal, then he becomes one with God even here. When all the knots of the heart are cut asunder, then the mortal becomes immortal, and he enjoys Brahman here." Here, on this earth, nowhere else.

A few words ought to be said here. You will generally hear that this Vedanta, this philosophy and other Eastern systems, look only to something beyond, letting go the enjoyments and struggle of this life. This idea is entirely wrong. It is only ignorant people who do not know anything of Eastern thought, and never had brain enough to understand anything of its real teaching, that tell you so. On the contrary, we read in our scriptures that our philosophers do not want to go to other worlds, but depreciate them as places where people weep and laugh for a little while only and then die. As long as we are weak we shall have to go through these experiences; but whatever is true, is here, and that is the human soul. And this also is insisted upon, that by committing suicide, we cannot escape the inevitable; we cannot evade it. But the right path is hard to find. The Hindu is just as practical as the Western, only we differ in our views of life. The one says, build a good house, let us have good clothes and food, intellectual culture, and so on, for this is the whole of life; and in that he is immensely practical. But the Hindu says, true knowledge of the world means knowledge of the soul, metaphysics; and he wants to enjoy that life. In America there was a great agnostic, a very noble man, a very good man, and a very fine speaker. He lectured on religion, which he said was of no use; why bother our heads about other worlds? He employed this simile; we have an orange here, and we want to squeeze all the juice out of it. I met him once and said, "I agree with you entirely. I have some fruit, and I too want to squeeze out the juice. Our difference lies in the choice of the fruit. You want an orange, and I prefer a mango. You think it is enough to live here and eat and drink and have a little scientific knowledge; but you have no right to say that that will suit all tastes. Such a conception is nothing to me. If I had only to learn how an apple falls to the ground, or how an electric current shakes my nerves, I would commit suicide. I want to understand the heart of things, the very kernel itself. Your study is the manifestation of life, mine is the life itself. My philosophy says you must know that and drive out from your mind all thoughts of heaven and hell and all other superstitions, even though they exist in the same sense that this world exists. I must know the heart of this life, its very essence, what it is, not only how it works and what are its manifestations. I want the why of everything, I leave the how to children. As one of your countrymen said, 'While I am smoking a cigarette, if I were to write a book, it would be the science of the cigarette.' It is good and great to be scientific, God bless them in their search; but when a man says that is all, he is talking foolishly, not caring to know the *raison d'être* of life, never studying existence itself. I may argue that all your knowledge is nonsense, without a basis. You are studying the manifestations of life, and when I ask you what life is, you say you do not know. You are welcome to your study, but leave me to mine."

I am practical, very practical, in my own way. So your idea that only the West is practical is nonsense. You are practical in one way, and I in another. There are different types of men and minds. If in the East a man is told that he will find out the truth by standing on one leg all his life, he will pursue that method. If in the West men hear that there is a gold mine somewhere in an uncivilised country, thousands will face the dangers there, in the hope of getting the gold; and, perhaps, only one succeeds. The same men have heard that they have souls but are content to leave the care of them to the church. The first man will not go near the savages, he says it may be dangerous. But if we tell him that on the top of a high mountain lives a wonderful sage who can give him knowledge of the soul, he tries to climb up to him, even if he be killed in the attempt. Both types of men are practical, but the mistake lies in regarding this world as the whole of life. Yours is the vanishing point of enjoyment of the senses — there is nothing permanent in it, it only brings more and more misery – while mine brings eternal peace.

I do not say your view is wrong, you are welcome to it. Great good and blessing come out of it, but do not, therefore, condemn my view. Mine also is practical in its own way. Let us all work on our own plans. Would to God all of us were equally practical on both sides. I have seen some scientists who were equally practical, both as scientists and as spiritual men, and it is my great hope that in course of time the whole of humanity will be efficient in the same manner. When a kettle of water is coming to the boil, if you watch the phenomenon, you find first one bubble rising, and then another and so on, until at last they all join, and a tremendous commotion takes place. This world is very similar. Each individual is like a bubble, and the nations, resemble many bubbles. Gradually these nations are joining, and I am sure the day will come when separation will vanish and that Oneness to which we are all going will become manifest. A time must come when every man will be as intensely practical in the scientific world as in the spiritual, and then that Oneness, the harmony of Oneness, will pervade the whole world. The whole of mankind will become Jivanmuktas – free whilst living. We are all struggling towards that one end through our jealousies and hatreds, through our love and co-operation. A tremendous stream is flowing towards the ocean carrying us all along with it; and though like straws and scraps of paper we may at times float aimlessly about, in the long run we are sure to join the Ocean of Life and Bliss.

❑

10

The Freedom of the Soul

(Delivered in London, 5th November 1896)

The Katha Upanishad, which we have been studying, was written much later than that to which we now turn – the Chhândogya. The language is more modern, and the thought more organised. In the older Upanishads the language is very archaic, like that of the hymn portion of the Vedas, and one has to wade sometimes through quite a mass of unnecessary things to get at the essential doctrines. The ritualistic literature about which I told you which forms the second division of the Vedas, has left a good deal of its mark upon this old Upanishad, so that more than half of it is still ritualistic. There is, however, one great gain in studying the very old Upanishads. You trace, as it were, the historical growth of spiritual ideas. In the more recent Upanishads, the spiritual ideas have been collected and brought into one place; as in the Bhagavad Gitâ, for instance, which we may, perhaps, look upon as the last of the Upanishads, you do not find any inkling of these ritualistic ideas. The Gita is like a bouquet composed of the beautiful flowers of spiritual truths collected from the Upanishads. But in the Gita you cannot study the rise of the spiritual ideas, you cannot trace them to their source. To do that, as has been pointed out by many, you must study the Vedas. The great idea of holiness that has been attached to these books has preserved them, more than any other book in the world, from mutilation. In them, thoughts at their highest and at their lowest have all been preserved, the essential and the non-essential, the most ennobling teachings and the simplest matters of detail stand side by side; for nobody has dared to touch them. Commentators came and tried to smooth them down and to bring out wonderful new ideas from the old things; they tried to find spiritual ideas in even the most ordinary statements, but the texts remained, and as such, they are the most wonderful historical study. We all know that in the scriptures of every religion changes were made to suit the growing spirituality of later times; one word was changed here and another put in there, and so on. This, probably, has not been done with the Vedic literature, or if ever done, it is almost imperceptible. So we have this great advantage, we are able to study thoughts in their original significance, to note how they developed, how from materialistic ideas finer and finer spiritual ideas are evolved, until they attained their greatest height in the Vedanta. Descriptions of some of the old manners and customs are also there, but they do not appear much in the Upanishads. The language used is peculiar, terse, mnemonic.

The writers of these books simply jotted down these lines as helps to remember certain facts which they supposed were already well known. In a narrative, perhaps, which they are telling, they take it for granted that it is well known to everyone they are addressing. Thus a great difficulty arises, we scarcely know the real meaning of any one of these stories, because the traditions have nearly died out, and the little that is left of them has been very much exaggerated. Many new interpretations have been put upon them, so that when you find them in the Purânas they have already become lyrical poems. Just as in the West, we find this prominent fact in the political development of Western races that they cannot bear absolute rule, that they are always trying to prevent any one man from ruling over them, and are gradually advancing to higher and higher democratic ideas, higher and higher ideas of physical liberty, so, in Indian metaphysics, exactly the same phenomenon appears in the development of spiritual life. The multiplicity of gods gave place to one God of the universe, and in the Upanishads there is a rebellion even against that one

God. Not only was the idea of many governors of the universe ruling their destinies unbearable, but it was also intolerable that there should be one person ruling this universe. This is the first thing that strikes us. The idea grows and grows, until it attains its climax. In almost all of the Upanishads, we find the climax coming at the last, and that is the dethroning of this God of the universe. The personality of God vanishes, the impersonality comes. God is no more a person, no more a human being, however magnified and exaggerated, who rules this universe, but He has become an embodied principle in every being, immanent in the whole universe. It would be illogical to go from the Personal God to the Impersonal, and at the same time to leave man as a person. So the personal man is broken down, and man as principle is built up. The person is only a phenomenon, the principle is behind it. Thus from both sides, simultaneously, we find the breaking down of personalities and the approach towards principles, the Personal God approaching the Impersonal, the personal man approaching the Impersonal Man. Then come the succeeding stages of the gradual convergence of the two advancing lines of the Impersonal God and the Impersonal Man. And the Upanishads embody the stages through which these two lines at last become one, and the last word of each Upanishad is, "Thou art That". There is but One Eternally Blissful Principle, and that One is manifesting Itself as all this variety.

Then came the philosophers. The work of the Upanishads seems to have ended at that point; the next was taken up by the philosophers. The framework was given them by the Upanishads, and they had to fill in the details. So, many questions would naturally arise. Taking for granted that there is but One Impersonal Principle which is manifesting Itself in all these manifold forms, how is it that the One becomes many? It is another way of putting the same old question which in its crude form comes into the human heart as the inquiry into the cause of evil and so forth. Why does evil exist in the world, and what is its cause? But the same question has now become refined, abstracted. No more is it asked from the platform of the senses why we are unhappy, but from the platform of philosophy. How is it that this One Principle becomes manifold? And the answer, as we have seen, the best answer that India has produced is the theory of Maya which says that It really has not become manifold, that It really has not lost any of Its real nature. Manifoldness is only apparent. Man is only apparently a person, but in reality he is the Impersonal Being. God is a person only apparently, but really He is the Impersonal Being.

Even in this answer there have been succeeding stages, and philosophers have varied in their opinions. All Indian philosophers did not admit this theory of Maya. Possibly most of them did not. There are dualists, with a crude sort of dualism, who would not allow the question to be asked, but stifled it at its very birth. They said, "You have no right to ask such a question, you have no right to ask for an explanation; it is simply the will of God, and we have to submit to it quietly. There is no liberty for the human soul. Everything is predestined – what we shall do, have, enjoy, and suffer; and when suffering comes, it is our duty to endure it patiently; if we do not, we shall be punished all the more. How do we know that? Because the Vedas say so." And thus they have their texts and their meanings and they want to enforce them.

There are others who, though not admitting the Maya theory, stand midway. They say that the whole of this creation forms, as it were, the body of God. God is the Soul of all souls and of the whole of nature. In the case of individual souls, contraction comes from evil doing. When a man does anything evil, his soul begins to contract and his power is diminished and goes on decreasing, until he does good works, when it expands again. One idea seems to be common in all the Indian systems, and I think, in every system in the world, whether they know it or not, and that is what I should call the divinity of man. There is no one system in the world, no real religion, which does not hold the idea that the human soul, whatever it be, or whatever its relation to God, is essentially pure and perfect, whether expressed in the language of mythology, allegory, or philosophy. Its real nature is blessedness and power, not weakness and misery. Somehow or other this misery has come. The crude systems may call it a personified evil, a devil, or an Ahriman, to explain how this misery came. Other systems may try to make a God and a devil in one, who makes some people miserable and others happy, without any reason whatever. Others again, more thoughtful, bring in the theory of Maya and so forth. But one fact stands out clearly, and it is with this that we have to deal. After all, these philosophical ideas and systems are but gymnastics of the mind, intellectual exercises. The one great idea that to me seems to be clear, and comes out through masses of superstition in every country and in every religion, is the one luminous idea that man is divine, that divinity is our nature.

Whatever else comes is a mere superimposition, as the Vedanta calls it. Something has been superimposed, but that divine nature never dies. In the most degraded as well as in the most saintly it is ever present. It has to be called out, and it will work itself out. We have to ask and it will manifest itself. The people of old knew that fire lived in the flint and in dry wood, but friction was necessary to call it out. So this fire of freedom and purity is the nature of every soul, and not a quality, because qualities can be acquired and therefore can be lost. The soul is one with Freedom, and the soul is one with Existence, and the soul is one with Knowledge. The Sat-Chit-Ânanda – Existence-Knowledge-Bliss Absolute – is the nature, the birthright of the Soul, and all the manifestations that we see are Its expressions, dimly or brightly manifesting Itself. Even death is but a manifestation of that Real Existence. Birth and death, life and decay, degeneration and regeneration – are all manifestations of that Oneness. So, knowledge, however it manifests itself, either as ignorance or as learning, is but the manifestation of that same Chit, the essence of knowledge; the difference is only in degree, and not in kind. The difference in knowledge between the lowest worm that crawls under our feet and the highest genius that the world may produce is only one of degree, and not of kind. The Vedantin thinker boldly says that the enjoyments in this life, even the most degraded joys, are but manifestations of that One Divine Bliss, the Essence of the Soul.

This idea seems to be the most prominent in Vedanta, and, as I have said, it appears to me that every religion holds it. I have yet to know the religion which does not. It is the one universal idea working through all religions. Take the Bible for instance. You find there the allegorical statement that the first man Adam was pure, and that his purity was obliterated by his evil deeds afterwards. It is clear from this allegory that they thought that the nature of the primitive man was perfect. The impurities that we see, the weaknesses that we feel, are but superimpositions on that nature, and the subsequent history of the Christian religion shows that they also believe in the possibility, nay, the certainty of regaining that old state. This is the whole history of the Bible, Old and New Testaments together. So with the Mohammedans: they also believed in Adam and the purity of Adam, and through Mohammed the way was opened to regain that lost state. So with the Buddhists: they believe in the state called Nirvana which is beyond this relative world. It is exactly the same as the Brahman of the Vedantins, and the whole system of the Buddhists is founded upon the idea of regaining that lost state of Nirvana. In every system we find this doctrine present, that you cannot get anything which is not yours already. You are indebted to nobody in this universe. You claim your own birthright, as it has been most poetically expressed by a great Vedantin philosopher, in the title of one of his books — "The attainment of our own empire". That empire is ours; we have lost it and we have to regain it. The Mâyâvâdin, however, says that this losing of the empire was a hallucination; you never lost it. This is the only difference.

Although all the systems agree so far that we had the empire, and that we have lost it, they give us varied advice as to how to regain it. One says that you must perform certain ceremonies, pay certain sums of money to certain idols, eat certain sorts of food, live in a peculiar fashion to regain that empire. Another says that if you weep and prostrate yourselves and ask pardon of some Being beyond nature, you will regain that empire. Again, another says if you love such a Being with all your heart, you will regain that empire. All this varied advice is in the Upanishads. As I go on, you will find it so. But the last and the greatest counsel is that you need not weep at all. You need not go through all these ceremonies, and need not take any notice of how to regain your empire, because you never lost it. Why should you go to seek for what you never lost? You are pure already, you are free already. If you think you are free, free you are this moment, and if you think you are bound, bound you will be. This is a very bold statement, and as I told you at the beginning of this course, I shall have to speak to you very boldly. It may frighten you now, but when you think over it, and realise it in your own life, then you will come to know that what I say is true. For, supposing that freedom is not your nature, by no manner of means can you become free. Supposing you were free and in some way you lost that freedom, that shows that you were not free to begin with. Had you been free, what could have made you lose it? The independent can never be made dependent; if it is really dependent, its independence was a hallucination.

Of the two sides, then, which will you take? If you say that the soul was by its own nature pure and free, it naturally follows that there was nothing in this universe which could make it bound or limited. But if there was anything in nature which could bind the soul, it naturally follows that it was not free, and your statement that it was free is a delusion. So if it is possible for us to attain to freedom, the conclusion is inevitable that the soul is by its nature free. It cannot be otherwise. Freedom means independence of anything outside, and that means that nothing outside itself could work upon it as a cause. The soul is causeless, and from this follow all the great ideas that we have. You cannot establish the immortality of the soul, unless you grant that it is by its nature free, or in other words, that it cannot be acted upon by anything outside. For death is an effect produced by some outside cause. I drink poison and I die, thus showing that my body can be acted upon by something outside that is called poison. But if it be true that the soul is free, it naturally follows that nothing can affect it, and it can never die. Freedom, immortality, blessedness, all depend upon the soul being beyond the law of causation, beyond this Maya. Of these two which will you take? Either make the first a delusion, or make the second a delusion. Certainly I will make the second a delusion. It is more consonant with all my feelings and aspirations. I am perfectly aware that I am free by nature, and I will not admit that this bondage is true and my freedom a delusion.

This discussion goes on in all philosophies, in some form or other. Even in the most modern philosophies you find the same discussion arising. There are two parties. One says that there is no soul, that the idea of soul is a delusion produced by the repeated transit of particles or matter, bringing about the combination which you call the body or brain; that the impression of freedom is the result of the vibrations and motions and continuous transit of these particles. There were Buddhistic sects who held the same view and illustrated it by this example: If young take a torch and whirl it round rapidly, there will be a circle of light. That circle does not really exist, because the torch is changing place every moment. We are but bundles of little particles, which in their rapid whirling produce the delusion of a permanent soul. The other party states that in the rapid succession of thought, matter occurs as a delusion, and does not really exist. So we see one side claiming that spirit is a delusion and the other, that matter is a delusion. Which side will you take? Of course, we will take the spirit and deny matter. The arguments are similar for both, only on the spirit side the argument is little stronger. For nobody has ever seen what matter is. We can only feel ourselves. I never knew a man who could feel matter outside of himself. Nobody was ever able to jump outside of himself. Therefore the argument is a little stronger on the side of the spirit. Secondly, the spirit theory explains the universe, whiles materialism does not. Hence the materialistic explanation is illogical. If you boil down all the philosophies and analyse them, you will find that they are reduced to one; or the other of these two positions. So here, too, in a more intricate form, in a more philosophical form, we find the same question about natural purity and freedom. Ones side says that the first is a delusion, and the other, that the second is a delusion. And, of course, we side with the second, in believing that our bondage is a delusion.

The solution of the Vedanta is that we are not bound, we are free already. Not only so, but to say or to think that we are bound is dangerous — it is a mistake, it is self-hypnotism. As soon as you say, "I am bound," "I am weak," "I am helpless," woe unto you; you rivet one more chain upon yourself. Do not say it, do not think it. I have heard of a man who lived in a forest and used to repeat day and night, "Shivoham" — I am the Blessed One — and one day a tiger fell upon him and dragged him away to kill him; people on the other side of the river saw it, and heard the voice so long as voice remained in him, saying, "Shivoham" — even in the very jaws of the tiger. There have been many such men. There have been cases of men who, while being cut to pieces, have blessed their enemies. "I am He, I am He; and so art thou. I am pure and perfect and so are all my enemies. You are He, and so am I." That is - the position of strength. Nevertheless, there are great and wonderful things in the religions of the dualists; wonderful is the idea of the Personal God apart from nature, whom we worship and love. Sometimes this idea is very soothing. But, says the Vedanta, the soothing is something like the effect that comes from an opiate, not natural. It brings weakness in the long run, and what this world wants today, more than it ever did before, is strength. It is weakness, says the Vedanta, which is the cause of all misery in this world. Weakness is the one cause of suffering. We become miserable because we are weak. We lie, steal, kill, and commit other crimes, because we are weak. We suffer because we are weak. We die because we are weak. Where there is nothing to weaken us, there is no death nor sorrow. We are miserable through delusion. Give up the delusion, and the whole thing vanishes. It is plain and simple indeed. Through all these philosophical discussions and tremendous mental gymnastics we come to this one religious idea, the simplest in the whole world.

The monistic Vedanta is the simplest form in which you can put truth. To teach dualism was a tremendous mistake made in India and elsewhere, because people did not look at the ultimate principles, but only thought of the process which is very intricate indeed. To many, these tremendous philosophical and logical propositions were alarming. They thought these things could not be made universal, could not be followed in everyday practical life, and that under the guise of such a philosophy much laxity of living would arise.

But I do not believe at all that monistic ideas preached to the world would produce immorality and weakness. On the contrary, I have reason to believe that it is the only remedy there is. If this be the truth, why let people drink ditch water when the stream of life is flowing by? If this be the truth, that they are all pure, why not at this moment teach it to the whole world? Why not teach it with the voice of thunder to every man that is born, to saints and sinners, men, women, and children, to the man on the throne and to the man sweeping the streets?

It appears now a very big and a very great undertaking; to many it appears very startling, but that is because of superstition, nothing else. By eating all sorts of bad and indigestible food, or by starving ourselves, we are incompetent to eat a good meal. We have listened to words of weakness from our childhood. You hear people say that they do not believe in ghosts, but at the same time, there are very few who do not get a little creepy sensation in the dark. It is simply superstition. So with all religious superstitions There are people in this country who, if I told them there was no such being as the devil, will think all religion is gone. Many people have said to me, how can there be religion without a devil? How can there be religion without someone to direct us? How can we live without being ruled by somebody? We like to be so treated, because we have become used to it. We are not happy until we feel we have been reprimanded by somebody every day. The same superstition! But however terrible it may seem now, the time will come when we shall look back, each one of us, and smile at every one of those superstitions which covered the pure and eternal soul, and repeat with gladness, with truth, and with strength, I am free, and was free, and always will be free. This monistic idea will come out of Vedanta, and it is the one idea that deserves to live. The scriptures may perish tomorrow. Whether this idea first flashed into the brains of Hebrews or of people living in the Arctic regions, nobody cares. For this is the truth and truth is eternal; and truth itself teaches that it is not the special property of any individual or nation. Men, animals, and gods are all common recipients of this one truth. Let them all receive it. Why make life miserable? Why let people fall into all sorts of superstitions? I will give ten thousand lives, if twenty of them will give up their superstition. Not only in this country, but in the land of its very birth, if you tell people this truth, they are frightened. They say, "This idea is for Sannyâsins who give up the world and live in forests; for them it is all right. But for us poor householders, we must all have some sort of fear, we must have ceremonies," and so on.

Dualistic ideas have ruled the world long enough, and this is the result. Why not make a new experiment? It may take ages for all minds to receive monism, but why not begin now? If we have told it to twenty persons in our lives, we have done a great work.

There is one idea which often militates against it. It is this. It is all very well to say, "I am the Pure, the Blessed," but I cannot show it always in my life. That is true; the ideal is always very hard. Every child that is born sees the sky overhead very far away, but is that any reason why we should not look towards the sky? Would it mend matters to go towards superstition? If we cannot get nectar, would it mend matters for us to drink poison? Would it be any help for us, because we cannot realise the truth immediately, to go into darkness and yield to weakness and superstition?

I have no objection to dualism in many of its forms. I like most of them, but I have objections to every form of teaching which inculcates weakness. This is the one question I put to every man, woman, or child, when they are in physical, mental, or spiritual training. Are you strong? Do you feel strength? – for I know it is truth alone that gives strength. I know that truth alone gives life, and nothing but going towards reality will make us strong, and none will reach truth until he is strong. Every system, therefore, which weakens the mind, makes one superstitious, makes one mope, makes one desire all sorts of wild impossibilities, mysteries, and superstitions, I do not like, because its effect is dangerous. Such systems never bring any good; such things create morbidity in the mind, make it weak, so weak that in course of time it will be almost impossible to receive truth or live up to it. Strength, therefore, is the one thing needful. Strength is the medicine for the world's disease. Strength is the medicine which the poor must have when tyrannised over by the rich. Strength is the medicine that the ignorant must have when oppressed by the learned; and it is the medicine that sinners must have when tyrannised over by other sinners; and nothing gives such strength as this idea of monism. Nothing makes us so moral as this idea of monism. Nothing makes us work so well at our best and highest as when all the responsibility is thrown upon ourselves. I challenge everyone of you. How will you behave if I put a little baby in your hands? Your whole life will be changed for the moment; whatever you may be, you must become selfless for the time being. You will give up all your criminal ideas as soon as responsibility is thrown upon you – your whole character will change. So if the whole responsibility is thrown upon our own shoulders, we shall be at our highest and best; when we have nobody to grope towards, no devil to lay our blame upon, no Personal God to carry our burdens, when we are alone responsible, then we shall rise to our highest and best. I am responsible for my fate, I am the bringer of good unto myself, I am the bringer of evil. I am the Pure and Blessed One. We must reject all thoughts that assert the contrary. "I have neither death nor fear, I have neither caste nor creed, I have neither father nor mother nor brother, neither friend nor foe, for I am Existence, Knowledge, and Bliss Absolute; I am the Blissful One, I am the Blissful One. I am not bound either by virtue or vice, by happiness or misery. Pilgrimages and books and ceremonials can never bind me. I have neither hunger nor thirst; the body is not mine, nor am I subject to the superstitions and decay that come to the body, I am Existence, Knowledge, and Bliss Absolute; I am the Blissful One, I am the Blissful One."

This, says the Vedanta, is the only prayer that we should have. This is the only way to reach the goal, to tell ourselves, and to tell everybody else, that we are divine. And as we go on repeating this, strength comes. He who falters at first will get stronger and stronger, and the voice will increase in volume until the truth takes possession of our hearts, and courses through our veins, and permeates our bodies. Delusion will vanish as the light becomes more and more effulgent, load after load of ignorance will vanish, and then will come a time when all else has disappeared and the Sun alone shines.

❑

11

The Cosmos: The Macrocosm

(Delivered in New York, 19th January 1896)

The flowers that we see all around us are beautiful, beautiful is the rising of the morning sun, beautiful are the variegated hues of nature. The whole universe is beautiful, and man has been enjoying it since his appearance on earth. Sublime and awe-inspiring are the mountains; the gigantic rushing rivers rolling towards the sea, the trackless deserts, the infinite ocean, the starry heavens – all these are awe-inspiring, sublime, and beautiful indeed. The whole mass of existence which we call nature has been acting on the human mind since time immemorial. It has been acting on the thought of man, and as its reaction has come out the question: What are these, whence are they? As far back as the time of the oldest portion of that most ancient human composition, the Vedas, we find the same question asked: "Whence is this? When there was neither aught nor naught, and darkness was hidden in darkness, who projected this universe? How? Who knows the secret?" And the question has come down to us at the present time. Millions of attempts have been made to answer it, yet millions of times it will have to be answered again. It is not that each answer was a failure; every answer to this question contained a part of truth, and this truth gathers strength as time rolls on. I will try to present before you the outline of the answer that I have gathered from the ancient philosophers of India; in harmony with modern knowledge.

We find that in this oldest of questions a few points had been already solved. The first is that there was a time when there was "neither aught nor naught", when this world did not exist; our mother earth with the seas and oceans, the rivers, and mountains, cities and villages human races, animals, plants, birds, and planets and luminaries, all this infinite variety of creation, had no existence. Are we sure of that? We will try to trace how this conclusion is arrived at. What does man see around him? Take a little plant. He puts a seed in the ground, and later, he finds a plant peep out, lift itself slowly above the ground, and grow and grow, till it becomes a gigantic tree. Then it dies, leaving only the seed. It completes the circle — it comes out of the seed, becomes the tree, and ends in the seed again. Look at a bird, how from the egg it springs, lives its life, and then dies, leaving other eggs, seeds of future birds. So with the animals, so with man. Everything in nature begins, as it were, from certain seeds, certain rudiments, certain fine forms, and becomes grosser and grosser, and develops, going on that way for a certain time, and then again goes back to that fine form, and subsides. The raindrop in which the beautiful sunbeam is playing was drawn in the form of vapour from the ocean, went far away into the air, and reached a region where it changed into water, and dropped down in its present form — to be converted into vapour again. So with everything in nature by which we are surrounded. We know that the huge mountains are being worked upon by glaciers and rivers, which are slowly but surely pounding them and pulverising them into sand, that drifts away into the ocean where it settles down on its bed, layer after layer, becoming hard as rocks, once more to be heaped up into mountains of a future generation. Again they will be pounded and pulverised, and thus the course goes on. From sand rise these mountains; unto sand they go.

If it be true that nature is uniform throughout, if it be true, and so far no human experience has contradicted it, that the same method under which a small grain of sand is created, works in creating the gigantic suns and stars and all this universe, if it be true that the whole of this universe is built on exactly the same plan as the atom, if it be true that the same law prevails throughout the universe, then, as it has been said in the Vedas, "Knowing one lump of clay we know the nature of all the clay that is in the universe." Take up a little plant and study its life, and we know the universe as it is. If we know one grain of sand, we understand the secret of the whole universe. Applying this course of reasoning to phenomena, we find, in the first place, that everything is almost similar at the beginning and the end. The mountain comes from the sand, and goes back to the sand; the river comes out of vapour, and goes back to vapour; plant life comes from the seed, and goes back to the seed; human life comes out of human germs, and goes back to human germs. The universe with its stars and planets has come out of a nebulous state and must go back to it. What do we learn from this? That the manifested or the grosser state is the effect, and the finer state the cause. Thousands of years ago, it was demonstrated by Kapila, the great father of all philosophy, that destruction means going back to the cause. If this table here is destroyed, it will go back to its cause, to those fine forms and particles which, combined, made this form which we call a table. If a man dies, he will go back to the elements which gave him his body; if this earth dies, it will go back to the elements which gave it form. This is what is called destruction, going back to the cause. Therefore we learn that the effect is the same as the cause, not different. It is only in another form. This glass is an effect, and it had its cause, and this cause is present in this form. A certain amount of the material called glass plus the force in the hands of the manufacturer, are the causes, the instrumental and the material, which, combined, produced this form called a glass. The force which was in the hands of the manufacturer is present in the glass as the power of adhesion, without which the particles would fall apart; and the glass material is also present. The glass is only a manifestation of these fine causes in a new shape, and if it be broken to pieces, the force which was present in the form of adhesion will go back and join its own element, and the particles of glass will remain the same until they take new forms.

Thus we find that the effect is never different from the cause. It is only that this effect is a reproduction of the cause in a grosser form. Next, we learn that all these particular forms which we call plants, animals, or men are being repeated *ad infinitum*, rising and falling. The seed produces the tree. The tree produces the seed, which again comes up as another tree, and so on and on; there is no end to it. Water-drops roll down the mountains into the ocean, and rise again as vapour, go back to the mountains and again come down to the ocean. So, rising and falling, the cycle goes on. So with all lives, so with all existence that we can see, feel, hear, or imagine. Everything that is within the bounds of our knowledge is proceeding in the same way, like breathing in and breathing out in the human body. Everything in creation goes on in this form, one wave rising, another falling, rising again, falling again. Each wave has its hollow, each hollow has its wave. The same law must apply to the universe taken as a whole, because of its uniformity. This universe must be resolved into its causes; the sun, moon, stars, and earth, the body and mind, and everything in this universe must return to their finer causes, disappear, be destroyed as it were. But they will live in the causes as fine forms. Out of these fine forms they will emerge again as new earths, suns, moons, and stars.

There is one fact more to learn about this rising and falling. The seed comes out of the tree; it does not immediately become a tree, but has a period of inactivity, or rather, a period of very fine unmanifested action. The seed has to work for some time beneath the soil. It breaks into pieces, degenerates as it were, and regeneration comes out of that degeneration. In the beginning, the whole of this universe has to work likewise for a period in that minute form, unseen and unmanifested, which is called chaos, and; out of that comes a new projection. The whole period of one manifestation of this universe — its going down into the finer form, remaining there for some time, and coming out again — is, in Sanskrit, called a Kalpa or a Cycle. Next comes a very important question especially for modern; times. We see that the finer forms develop slowly and slowly, and gradually becomes grosser and grosser. We have seen that the cause is the same as the effect, and the effect is only the cause in another form. Therefore this whole universe cannot be produced out of nothing. Nothing comes without a cause, and the cause is the effect in another form.

Out of what has this universe been produced then? From a preceding fine universe. Out of what has men been produced? The preceding fine form. Out of what has the tree been produced? Out of the seed; the whole of the tree was there in the seed. It comes out and becomes manifest. So, the whole of this universe has been created out of this very universe existing in a minute form. It has been made manifest now. It will go back to that minute form, and again will be made manifest. Now we find that the fine forms slowly come out and become grosser and grosser until they reach their limit, and when they reach their limit they go back further and further, becoming finer and finer again. This coming out of the fine and becoming gross, simply changing the arrangements of its parts, as it were, is what in modern times called evolution. This is very true, perfectly true; we see it in our lives. No rational man can possibly quarrel with these evolutionists. But we have to learn one thing more. We have to go one step further, and what is that? That every evolution is preceded by an involution. The seed is the father of the tree, but another tree was itself the father of the seed. The seed is the fine form out of which the big tree comes, and another big tree was the form which is involved in that seed. The whole of this universe was present in the cosmic fine universe. The little cell, which becomes afterwards the man, was simply the involved man and becomes evolved as a man. If this is clear, we have no quarrel with the evolutionists, for we see that if they admit this step, instead of their destroying religion, they will be the greatest supporters of it.

We see then, that nothing can be created out of nothing. Everything exists through eternity, and will exist through eternity. Only the movement is in succeeding waves and hollows, going back to fine forms, and coming out into gross manifestations. This involution and evolution is going on throughout the whole of nature. The whole series of evolution beginning with the lowest manifestation of life and reaching up to the highest, the most perfect man, must have been the involution of something else. The question is: The involution of what? What was involved? God. The evolutionist will tell you that your idea that it was God is wrong. Why? Because you see God is intelligent, but we find that intelligence develops much later on in the course of evolution. It is in man and the higher animals that we find intelligence, but millions of years have passed in this world before this intelligence came. This objection of the evolutionists does not hold water, as we shall see by applying our theory. The tree comes out of the seed, goes back to the seed; the beginning and the end are the same. The earth comes out of its cause and returns to it. We know that if we can find the beginning we can find the end. *E converso*, if we find the end we can find the beginning. If that is so, take this whole evolutionary series, from the protoplasm at one end to the perfect man at the other, and this whole series is one life. In the end we find the perfect man, so in the beginning it must have been the same. Therefore, the protoplasm was the involution of the highest intelligence. You may not see it but that involved intelligence is what is uncoiling itself until it becomes manifested in the most perfect man. That can be mathematically demonstrated. If the law of conservation of energy is true, you cannot get anything out of a machine unless you put it in there first. The amount of work that you get out of an engine is exactly the same as you have put into it in the form of water and coal, neither more nor less. The work I am doing now is just what I put into me, in the shape of air, food, and other things. It is only a question of change and manifestation. There cannot be added in the economy of this universe one particle of matter or one foot-pound of force, nor can one particle of matter or one foot-pound of force be taken out. If that be the case, what is this intelligence? If it was not present in the protoplasm, it must have come all of a sudden, something coming out of nothing, which is absurd. It, therefore, follows absolutely that the perfect man, the free man, the God-man, who has gone beyond the laws of nature, and transcended everything, who has no more to go through this process of evolution, through birth and death, that man called the "Christ-man" by the Christians, and the "Buddha-man" by the Buddhists, and the "Free" by the Yogis — that perfect man who is at one end of the chain of evolution was involved in the cell of the protoplasm, which is at the other end of the same chain.

Applying the same reason to the whole of the universe, we see that intelligence must be the Lord of creation, the cause. What is the most evolved notion that man has of this universe? It is intelligence, the adjustment of part to part, the display of intelligence, of which the ancient design theory was an attempt at expression. The beginning was, therefore, intelligence. At the beginning that intelligence becomes involved, and in the end that intelligence gets evolved. The sum total of the intelligence displayed in the universe must, therefore, be the involved universal intelligence unfolding itself. This universal intelligence is what we call God. Call it by any other name, it is absolutely certain that in the beginning there is that Infinite cosmic intelligence. This cosmic intelligence gets involved, and it manifests, evolves itself, until it becomes the perfect man, the "Christ-man," the "Buddha-man." Then it goes back to its own source. That is why all the scriptures say, "In Him we live and move and have our being." That is why all the scriptures preach that we come from God and go back to God. Do not be frightened by theological terms; if terms frighten you, you are not fit to be philosophers. This cosmic intelligence is what the theologians call God.

I have been asked many times, "Why do you use that old word, God? " Because it is the best word for our purpose; you cannot find a better word than that, because all the hopes, aspirations, and happiness of humanity have been centred in that word. It is impossible now to change the word. Words like these were first coined by great saints who realised their import and understood their meaning. But as they become current in society, ignorant people take these words, and the result is that they lose their spirit and glory. The word God has been used from time immemorial, and the idea of this cosmic intelligence, and all that is great and holy, is associated with it. Do you mean to say that because some fool says it is not all right, we should throw it away? Another man may come and say, "Take *my* word," and another again, "Take *my* word." So there will be no end to foolish words. Use the old word, only use it in the true spirit, cleanse it of superstition, and realise fully what this great ancient word means. If you understand the power of the laws of association, you will know that these words are associated with innumerable majestic and powerful ideas; they have been used and worshipped by millions of human souls and associated by them with all that is highest and best, all that is rational, all that is lovable, and all that is great and grand in human nature. And they come as suggestions of these associations, and cannot be given up. If I tried to express all these by only telling you that God created the universe, it would have conveyed no meaning to you. Yet, after all this struggle, we have come back to Him, the Ancient and Supreme One.

We now see that all the various forms of cosmic energy, such as matter, thought, force, intelligence and so forth, are simply the manifestations of that cosmic intelligence, or, as we shall call it henceforth, the Supreme Lord. Everything that you see, feel, or hear, the whole universe, is His creation, or to be a little more accurate, is His projection; or to be still more accurate, is the Lord Himself. It is He who is shining as the sun and the stars, He is the mother earth. He is the ocean Himself. He comes as gentle showers, He is the gentle air that we breathe in, and He it is who is working as force in the body. He is the speech that is uttered, He is the man who is talking. He is the audience that is here. He is the platform on which I stand, He is the light that enables me to see your faces. It is all He. He Himself is both the material and the efficient cause of this universe, and He it is that gets involved in the minute cell, and evolves at the other end and becomes God again. He it is that comes down and becomes the lowest atom, and slowly unfolding His nature, rejoins Himself. This is the mystery of the universe. "Thou art the man, Thou art the woman, Thou art the strong man walking in the pride of youth, Thou art the old man tottering on crutches, Thou art in everything. Thou art everything, O Lord." This is the only solution of the Cosmos that satisfies the human intellect. In one word, we are born of Him, we live in Him, and unto Him we return.

❑

12

The Cosmos: The Microcosm

(Delivered in New York, 26th January 1896)

The human mind naturally wants to get outside, to peer out of the body, as it were, through the channels of the organs. The eye must see, the ear must hear, the senses must sense the external world – and naturally the beauties and sublimities of nature captivate the attention of man first. The first questions that arose in the human soul were about the external world. The solution of the mystery was asked of the sky, of the stars, of the heavenly bodies, of the earth, of the rivers, of the mountains, of the ocean; and in all ancient religions we find traces of how the groping human mind at first caught at everything external. There was a river-god, a sky-god, a cloud-god, a rain-god; everything external, all of which we now call the powers of nature, became metamorphosed, transfigured, into wills, into gods, into heavenly messengers. As the question went deeper and deeper, these external manifestations failed to satisfy the human mind, and finally the energy turned inward, and the question was asked of man's own soul. From the macrocosm the question was reflected back to the microcosm; from the external world the question was reflected to the internal. From analysing the external nature, man is led to analyse the internal; this questioning of the internal man comes with a higher state of civilisation, with a deeper insight into nature, with a higher state of growth.

The subject of discussion this afternoon is this internal man. No question is so near and dear to man's heart as that of the internal man. How many millions of times, in how many countries has this question been asked! Sages and kings, rich and poor, saints and sinners, every man, every woman, all have from time to time asked this question. Is there nothing permanent in this evanescent human life? Is there nothing, they have asked, which does not die away when this body dies? Is there not something living when this frame crumbles into dust? Is there not something which survives the fire which burns the body into ashes? And if so, what is its destiny? Where does it go? Whence did it come? These questions have been asked again and again, and so long as this creation lasts, so long as there are human brains to think, this question will have to be asked. Yet, it is not that the answer did not come; each time the answer came, and as time rolls on, the answer will gain strength more and more. The question was answered once for all thousands of years ago, and through all subsequent time it is being restated, reillustrated, made clearer to our intellect. What we have to do, therefore, is to make a restatement of the answer. We do not pretend to throw any new light on those all-absorbing problems, but only to put before you the ancient truth in the language of modern times, to speak the thoughts of the ancients in the language of the moderns, to speak the thoughts of the philosophers in the language of the people, to speak the thoughts of the angels in the language of man, to speak the thoughts of God in the language of poor humanity, so that man will understand them; for the same divine essence from which the ideas emanated is ever present in man, and, therefore, he can always understand them.

I am looking at you. How many things are necessary for this vision? First, the eyes. For if I am perfect in every other way, and yet have no eyes, I shall not be able to see you. Secondly, the real organ of vision. For the eyes are not the organs. They are but the instruments of vision, and behind them is the real organ, the nerve centre in the brain. If that centre be injured, a man may have the clearest pair of eyes, yet he will not be able to see anything. So, it is necessary that this centre, or the real organ, be there. Thus, with all our senses. The external ear is but the instrument for carrying the vibration of sound inward to the centre. Yet, that is not sufficient. Suppose in your library you are intently reading a book, and the clock strikes, yet you do not hear it. The sound is there, the pulsations in the air are there, the ear and the centre are also there, and these vibrations have been carried through the ear to the centre, and yet you do not hear it. What is wanting? The mind is not there. Thus we see that the third thing necessary is, that the mind must be there. First the external instruments, then the organ to which this external instrument will carry the sensation, and lastly the organ itself must be joined to the mind. When the mind is not joined to the organ, the organ and the ear may take the impression, and yet we shall not be conscious of it. The mind, too, is only the carrier; it has to carry the sensation still forward, and present it to the intellect. The intellect is the determining faculty and decides upon what is brought to it. Still this is not sufficient. The intellect must carry it forward and present the whole thing before the ruler in the body, the human soul, the king on the throne. Before him this is presented, and then from him comes the order, what to do or what not to do; and the order goes down in the same sequence to the intellect, to the mind, to the organs, and the organs convey it to the instruments, and the perception is complete.

The instruments are in the external body, the gross body of man; but the mind and the intellect are not. They are in what is called in Hindu philosophy the finer body; and what in Christian theology you read of as the spiritual body of man; finer, very much finer than the body, and yet not the soul. This soul is beyond them all. The external body perishes in a few years; any simple cause may disturb and destroy it. The finer body is not so easily perishable; yet it sometimes degenerates, and at other times becomes strong. We see how, in the old man, the mind loses its strength, how, when the body is vigorous, the mind becomes vigorous, how various medicines and drugs affect it, how everything external acts on it, and how it reacts on the external world. Just as the body has its progress and decadence, so also has the mind, and, therefore, the mind is not the soul, because the soul can neither decay nor degenerate. How can we know that? How can we know that there is something behind this mind? Because knowledge which is self-illuminating and the basis of intelligence cannot belong to dull, dead matter. Never was seen any gross matter which had intelligence as its own essence. No dull or dead matter can illumine itself. It is intelligence that illumines all matter. This hall is here only through intelligence because, as a hall, its existence would be unknown unless some intelligence built it. This body is not self-luminous; if it were, it would be so in a dead man also. Neither can the mind nor the spiritual body be self-luminous. They are not of the essence of intelligence. That which is self-luminous cannot decay. The luminosity of that which shines through a borrowed light comes and goes; but that which is light itself, what can make that come and go, flourish and decay? We see that the moon waxes and wanes, because it shines through the borrowed light of the sun. If a lump of iron is put into the fire and made red-hot, it glows and shines, but its light will vanish, because it is borrowed. So, decadence is possible only of that light which is borrowed and is not of its own essence.

Now we see that the body, the external shape, has no light as its own essence, is not self-luminous, and cannot know itself; neither can the mind. Why not? Because the mind waxes and wanes, because it is vigorous at one time and weak at another, because it can be acted upon by anything and everything. Therefore the light which shines through the mind is not its own. Whose is it then? It must belong to that which has it as its own essence, and as such, can never decay or die, never become stronger or weaker; it is self-luminous, it is luminosity itself. It cannot be that the soul knows, it *is* knowledge. It cannot be that the soul has existence, but it is existence. It cannot be that the soul is happy, it is happiness itself. That which is happy has borrowed its happiness; that which has knowledge has received its knowledge; and that which has relative existence has only a reflected existence. Wherever there are qualities these qualities have been reflected upon the substance, but the soul has not knowledge, existence, and blessedness as its qualities, they are the essence of the soul.

Again, it may be asked, why shall we take this for granted? Why shall we admit that the soul has knowledge, blessedness, existence, as its essence, and has not borrowed them? It may be argued, why not say that the soul's luminosity, the soul's blessedness, the soul's knowledge, are borrowed in the same way as the luminosity of the body is borrowed from the mind? The fallacy of arguing in this way will be that there will be no limit. From whom were these borrowed? If we say from some other source, the same question will be asked again. So, at last we shall have to come to one who is self-luminous; to make matters short then, the logical way is to stop where we get self-luminosity, and proceed no further.

We see, then, that this human being is composed first of this external covering, the body; secondly, the finer body, consisting of mind, intellect, and egoism. Behind them is the real Self of man. We have seen that all the qualities and powers of the gross body are borrowed from the mind, and the mind, the finer body, borrows its powers and luminosity from the soul, standing behind.

A great many questions now arise about the nature of this soul. If the existence of the soul is drawn from the argument that it is self-luminous, that knowledge, existence, blessedness are its essence, it naturally follows that this soul cannot have been created. A self-luminous existence, independent of any other existence, could never have been the outcome of anything. It always existed; there was never a time when it did not exist, because if the soul did not exist, where was time? Time is in the soul; it is when the soul reflects its powers on the mind and the mind thinks, that time comes. When there was no soul, certainly there was no thought, and without thought, there was no time. How can the soul, therefore, be said to be existing in time, when time itself exists in the soul? It has neither birth nor death, but it is passing through all these various stages. It is manifesting slowly and gradually from lower to higher, and so on. It is expressing its own grandeur, working through the mind on the body; and through the body it is grasping the external world and understanding it. It takes up a body and uses it; and when that body has failed and is used up, it takes another body; and so on it goes.

Here comes a very interesting question, that question which is generally known as the reincarnation of the soul. Sometimes people get frightened at the idea, and superstition is so strong that thinking men even believe that they are the outcome of nothing, and then, with the grandest logic, try to deduce the theory that although they have come out of zero, they will be eternal ever afterwards. Those that come out of zero will certainly have to go back to zero. Neither you, nor I nor anyone present, has come out of zero, nor will go back to zero. We have been existing eternally, and will exist, and there is no power under the sun or above the sun which can undo your or my existence or send us back to zero. Now this idea of reincarnation is not only not a frightening idea, but is most essential for the moral well-being of the human race. It is the only logical conclusion that thoughtful men can arrive at. If you are going to exist in eternity hereafter, it must be that you have existed through eternity in the past: it cannot be otherwise. I will try to answer a few objections that are generally brought against the theory. Although many of you will think they are very silly objections, still we have to answer them, for sometimes we find that the most thoughtful men are ready to advance the silliest ideas. Well has it been said that there never was an idea so absurd that it did not find philosophers to defend it. The first objection is, why do we not remember our past? Do we remember all our past in this life? How many of you remember what you did when you were babies? None of you remember your early childhood, and if upon memory depends your existence, then this argument proves that you did not exist as babies, because you do not remember your babyhood. It is simply unmitigated nonsense to say that our existence depends on our remembering it. Why should we remember the past? That brain is gone, broken into pieces, and a new brain has been manufactured. What has come to this brain is the resultant, the sum total of the impressions acquired in our past, with which the mind has come to inhabit the new body.

I, as I stand here, am the effect, the result, of all the infinite past which is tacked on to me. And why is it necessary for me to remember all the past? When a great ancient sage, a seer, or a prophet of old, who came face to face with the truth, says something, these modern men stand up and say, "Oh, he was a fool!" But just use another name, "Huxley says it, or Tyndall"; then it must be true, and they take it for granted. In place of ancient superstitions they have erected modern superstitions, in place of the old Popes of religion they have installed modern Popes of science. So we see that this objection as to memory is not valid, and that is about the only serious objection that is raised against this theory. Although we have seen that it is not necessary for the theory that there shall be the memory of past lives, yet at the same time, we are in a position to assert that there are instances which show that this memory does come, and that each one of us will get back this memory in that life in which he will become free. Then alone you will find that this world is but a dream; then alone you will realise in the soul of your soul that you are but actors and the world is a stage; then alone will the idea of non-attachment come to you with the power of thunder; then all this thirst for enjoyment, this clinging on to life and this world will vanish for ever; then the mind will see dearly as daylight how many times all these existed for you, how many millions of times you had fathers and mothers, sons and daughters, husbands and wives, relatives and friends, wealth and power. They came and went. How many times you were on the topmost crest of the wave, and how many times you were down at the bottom of despair! When memory will bring all these to you, then alone will you stand as a hero and smile when the world frowns upon you. Then alone will you stand up and say. "I care not for thee even, O Death, what terrors hast thou for me?" This will come to all.

Are there any arguments, any rational proofs for this reincarnation of the soul? So far we have been giving the negative side, showing that the opposite arguments to disprove it are not valid. Are there any positive proofs? There are; and most valid ones, too. No other theory except that of reincarnation accounts for the wide divergence that we find between man and man in their powers to acquire knowledge. First, let us consider the process by means of which knowledge is acquired. Suppose I go into the street and see a dog. How do I know it is a dog? I refer it to my mind, and in my mind are groups of all my past experiences, arranged and pigeon-holed, as it were. As soon as a new impression comes, I take it up and refer it to some of the old pigeon-holes, and as soon as I find a group of the same impressions already existing, I place it in that group, and I am satisfied. I know it is a dog, because it coincides with the impressions already there. When I do not find the cognates of this new experience inside, I become dissatisfied. When, not finding the cognates of an impression, we become dissatisfied, this state of the mind is called "ignorance"; but, when, finding the cognates of an impression already existing, we become satisfied, this is called "knowledge". When one apple fell, men became dissatisfied. Then gradually they found out the group. What was the group they found? That all apples fell, so they called it "gravitation". Now we see that without a fund of already existing experience, any new experience would be impossible, for there would be nothing to which to refer the new impression. So, if, as some of the European philosophers think, a child came into the world with what they call *tabula rasa*, such a child would never attain to any degree of intellectual power, because he would have nothing to which to refer his new experiences. We see that the power of acquiring knowledge varies in each individual, and this shows that each one of us has come with his own fund of knowledge. Knowledge can only be got in one way, the way of experience; there is no other way to know. If we have not experienced it in this life, we must have experienced it in other lives. How is it that the fear of death is everywhere? A little chicken is just out of an egg and an eagle comes, and the chicken flies in fear to its mother. There is an old explanation (I should hardly dignify it by such a name). It is called instinct. What makes that little chicken just out of the egg afraid to die? How is it that as soon as a duckling hatched by a hen comes near water, it jumps into it and swims? It never swam before, nor saw anything swim. People call it instinct. It is a big word, but it leaves us where we were before. Let us study this phenomenon of instinct. A child begins to play on the piano. At first she must pay attention to every key she is fingering, and as she goes on and on for months and years, the playing becomes almost involuntary, instinctive. What was first done with conscious will does not require later on an effort of the will. This is not yet a complete proof. One half remains, and that is that almost all the actions which are now instinctive can be brought under the control of the will. Each muscle of the body can be brought under control. This is perfectly well known. So the proof is complete by this double method, that what we now call instinct is degeneration of voluntary actions; therefore, if the analogy applies to the whole of creation, if all nature is uniform, then what is instinct in lower animals, as well as in men, must be the degeneration of will.

Applying the law we dwelt upon under macrocosm that each involution presupposes an evolution, and each evolution an involution, we see that instinct is involved reason. What we call instinct in men or animals must therefore be involved, degenerated, voluntary actions, and voluntary actions are impossible without experience. Experience started that knowledge, and that knowledge is there. The fear of death, the duckling taking to the water and all involuntary actions in the human being which have become instinctive, are the results of past experiences. So far we have proceeded very clearly, and so far the latest science is with us. But here comes one more difficulty. The latest scientific men are coming back to the ancient sages, and as far as they have done so, there is perfect agreement. They admit that each man and each animal is born with a fund of experience, and that all these actions in the mind are the result of past experience. "But what," they ask, "is the use of saying that that experience belongs to the soul? Why not say it belongs to the body, and the body alone? Why not say it is hereditary transmission?" This is the last question. Why not say that all the experience with which I am born is the resultant effect of all the past experience of my ancestors? The sum total of the experience from the little protoplasm up to the highest human being is in me, but it has come from body to body in the course of hereditary transmission. Where will the difficulty be? This question is very nice, and we admit some part of this hereditary transmission. How far? As far as furnishing the material. We, by our past actions, conform ourselves to a certain birth in a certain body, and the only suitable material for that body comes from the parents who have made themselves fit to have that soul as their offspring.

The simple hereditary theory takes for granted the most astonishing proposition without any proof, that mental experience can be recorded in matters, that mental experience can be involved in matter. When I look at you in the lake of my mind there is a wave. That wave subsides, but it remains in fine form, as an impression. We understand a physical impression remaining in the body. But what proof is there for assuming that the mental impression can remain in the body, since the body goes to pieces? What carries it? Even granting it were possible for each mental impression to remain in the body, that every impression, beginning from the first man down to my father, was in my father's body, how could it be transmitted to me? Through the bioplasmic cell? How could that be? Because the father's body does not come to the child *in toto*. The same parents may have a number of children; then, from this theory of hereditary transmission, where the impression and the impressed (that is to say, material) are one, it rigorously follows that by the birth of every child the parents must lose a part of their own impressions, or, if the parents should transmit the whole of their impressions, then, after the birth of the first child, their minds would be a vacuum.

Again, if in the bioplasmic cell the infinite amount of impressions from all time has entered, where and how is it? This is a most impossible position, and until these physiologists can prove how and where those impressions live in that cell, and what they mean by a mental impression sleeping in the physical cell, their position cannot be taken for granted. So far it is clear then, that this impression is in the mind, that the mind comes to take its birth and rebirth, and uses the material which is most proper for it, and that the mind which has made itself fit for only a particular kind of body will have to wait until it gets that material. This we understand. The theory then comes to this, that there is hereditary transmission so far as furnishing the material to the soul is concerned. But the soul migrates and manufactures body after body, and each thought we think, and each deed we do, is stored in it in fine forms, ready to spring up again and take a new shape. When I look at you a wave rises in my mind. It dives down, as it were, and becomes finer and finer, but it does not die. It is ready to start up again as a wave in the shape of memory. So all these impressions are in my mind, and when I die the resultant force of them will be upon me. A ball is here, and each one of us takes a mallet in his hands and strikes the ball from all sides; the ball goes from point to point in the room, and when it reaches the door it flies out. What does it carry out with it? The resultant of all these blows. That will give it its direction. So, what directs the soul when the body dies? The resultant, the sum total of all the works it has done, of the thoughts it has thought. If the resultant is such that it has to manufacture a new body for further experience, it will go to those parents who are ready to supply it with suitable material for that body. Thus, from body to body it will go, sometimes to a heaven, and back again to earth, becoming man, or some lower animal. This way it will go on until it has finished its experience, and completed the circle. It then knows its own nature, knows what it is, and ignorance vanishes, its powers become manifest, it becomes perfect; no more is there any necessity for the soul to work through physical bodies, nor is there any necessity for it to work through finer, or mental bodies. It shines in its own light, and is free, no more to be born, no more to die.

We will not go now into the particulars of this. But I will bring before you one more point with regard to this theory of reincarnation. It is the theory that advances the freedom of the human soul. It is the one theory that does not lay the blame of all our weakness upon somebody else, which is a common human fallacy. We do not look at our own faults; the eyes do not see themselves, they see the eyes of everybody else. We human beings are very slow to recognise our own weakness, our own faults, so long as we can lay the blame upon somebody else. Men in general lay all the blame of life on their fellow-men, or, failing that, on God, or they conjure up a ghost, and say it is fate. Where is fate, and who is fate? We reap what we sow. We are the makers of our own fate. None else has the blame, none has the praise. The wind is blowing; those vessels whose sails are unfurled catch it, and go forward on their way, but those which have their sails furled do not catch the wind. Is that the fault of the wind? Is it the fault of the merciful Father, whose wind of mercy is blowing without ceasing, day and night, whose mercy knows no decay, is it His fault that some of us are happy and some unhappy? We make our own destiny. His sun shines for the weak as well as for the strong. His wind blows for saint and sinner alike. He is the Lord of all, the Father of all, merciful, and impartial. Do you mean to say that He, the Lord of creation, looks upon the petty things of our life in the same light as we do? What a degenerate idea of God that would be! We are like little puppies, making life-and-death struggles here, and foolishly thinking that even God Himself will take it as seriously as we do. He knows what the puppies' play means. Our attempts to lay the blame on Him, making Him the punisher, and the rewarder, are only foolish. He neither punishes, nor rewards any. His infinite mercy is open to every one, at all times, in all places, under all conditions, unfailing, unswerving. Upon us depends how we use it. Upon us depends how we utilise it. Blame neither man, nor God, nor anyone in the world. When you find yourselves suffering, blame yourselves, and try to do better.

This is the only solution of the problem. Those that blame others — and, alas! the number of them is increasing every day — are generally miserable with helpless brains; they have brought themselves to that pass through their own mistakes and blame others, but this does not alter their position. It does not serve them in any way. This attempt to throw the blame upon others only weakens them the more. Therefore, blame none for your own faults, stand upon your own feet, and take the whole responsibility upon yourselves. Say, "This misery that I am suffering is of my own doing, and that very thing proves that it will have to be undone by me alone." That which I created, I can demolish; that which is created by some one else I shall never be able to destroy. Therefore, stand up, be bold, be strong. Take the whole responsibility on your own shoulders, and know that you are the creator of your own destiny. All the strength and succour you want is within yourselves. Therefore, make your own future. "Let the dead past bury its dead." The infinite future is before you, and you must always remember that each word, thought, and deed, lays up a store for you and that as the bad thoughts and bad works are ready to spring upon you like tigers, so also there is the inspiring hope that the good thoughts and good deeds are ready with the power of a hundred thousand angels to defend you always and for ever.

❑

13

Immortality

(Delivered in America)

What question has been asked a greater number of times, what idea has led men more to search the universe for an answer, what question is nearer and dearer to the human heart, what question is more inseparably connected with our existence, than this one, the immortality of the human soul? It has been the theme of poets and sages, of priests and prophets; kings on the throne have discussed it, beggars in the street have dreamt of it. The best of humanity have approached it, and the worst of men have hoped for it. The interest in the theme has not died yet, nor will it die so long as human nature exists. Various answers have been presented to the world by various minds. Thousands, again, in every period of history have given up the discussion, and yet the question remains fresh as ever. Often in the turmoil and struggle of our lives we seem to forget it, but suddenly some one dies – one, perhaps, whom we loved, one near and dear to our hearts is snatched away from us – and the struggle, the din and turmoil of the world around us, cease for a moment, and the soul asks the old questions "What after this?" "What becomes of the soul?"

All human knowledge proceeds out of experience; we cannot know anything except by experience. All our reasoning is based upon generalised experience, all our knowledge is but harmonised experience. Looking around us, what do we find? A continuous change. The plant comes out of the seed, grows into the tree, completes the circle, and comes back to the seed. The animal comes, lives a certain time, dies, and completes the circle. So does man. The mountains slowly but surely crumble away, the rivers slowly but surely dry up, rains come out of the sea, and go back to the sea. Everywhere circles are being completed, birth, growth, development, and decay following each other with mathematical precision. This is our everyday experience. Inside of it all, behind all this vast mass of what we call life, of millions of forms and shapes, millions upon millions of varieties, beginning from the lowest atom to the highest spiritualised man, we find existing a certain unity. Every day we find that the wall that was thought to be dividing one thing and another is being broken down, and all matter is coming to be recognised by modern science as one substance, manifesting in different ways and in various forms; the one life that runs through all like a continuous chain, of which all these various forms represent the links, link after link, extending almost infinitely, but of the same one chain. This is what is called evolution. It is an old, old idea, as old as human society, only it is getting fresher and fresher as human knowledge is progressing. There is one thing more, which the ancients perceived, but which in modern times is not yet so clearly perceived, and that is involution. The seed is becoming the plant; a grain of sand never becomes a plant. It is the father that becomes a child; a lump of clay never becomes the child. From what does this evolution come, is the question. What was the seed? It was the same as the tree. All the possibilities of a future tree are in that seed; all the possibilities of a future man are in the little baby; all the possibilities of any future life are in the germ. What is this? The ancient philosophers of India called it involution. We find then, that every evolution presupposes an involution. Nothing can be evolved which is not already there. Here, again, modern science comes to our help. You know by mathematical reasoning that the sum total of the energy that is displayed in the universe is the same throughout. You cannot take away one atom of matter or one foot-pound of force. You cannot add to the universe one atom of matter or one foot-pound of force. As such, evolution does not come out of zero; then, where does it come from? From previous involution. The child is the man involved, and the man is the child evolved.

The seed is the tree involved, and the tree is the seed evolved. All the possibilities of life are in the germ. The problem becomes a little clearer. Add to it the first idea of continuation of life. From the lowest protoplasm to the most perfect human being there is really but one life. Just as in one life we have so many various phases of expression, the protoplasm developing into the baby, the child, the young man, the old man, so, from that protoplasm up to the most perfect man we get one continuous life, one chain. This is evolution, but we have seen that each evolution presupposes an involution. The whole of this life which slowly manifests itself evolves itself from the protoplasm to the perfected human being — the Incarnation of God on earth — the whole of this series is but one life, and the whole of this manifestation must have been involved in that very protoplasm. This whole life, this very God on earth, was involved in it and slowly came out, manifesting itself slowly, slowly, slowly. The highest expression must have been there in the germ state in minute form; therefore this one force, this whole chain, is the involution of that cosmic life which is everywhere. It is this one mass of intelligence which, from the protoplasm up to the most perfected man, is slowly and slowly uncoiling itself. Not that it grows. Take off all ideas of growth from your mind. With the idea of growth is associated something coming from outside, something extraneous, which would give the lie to the truth that the Infinite which lies latent in every life is independent of all external conditions. It can never grow; It was always there, and only manifests Itself.

The effect is the cause manifested. There is no essential difference between the effect and the cause. Take this glass, for instance. There was the material, and the material plus the will of the manufacturer made the glass and these two were its causes and are present in it. In what form is the will present? As adhesion. If the force were not here, each particle would fall away. What is the effect then? It is the same as the cause, only taking; different form, a different composition. When the cause is changed and limited for a time, it becomes the effect We must remember this. Applying it to our idea of life the whole of the manifestation of this one series, from the protoplasm up to the most perfect man, must be the very same thing as cosmic life. First it got involved and became finer; and out of that fine something, which wet the cause, it has gone on evolving, manifesting itself, and becoming grosser.

But the question of immortality is not yet settled. We have seen that everything in this universe is indestructible. There is nothing new; there will be nothing new. The same series of manifestations are presenting themselves alternately like a wheel, coming up and going down. All motion in this universe is in the form of waves, successively rising and falling. Systems after systems are coming out of fine forms, evolving themselves, and taking grosser forms, again melting down, as it were, and going back to the fine forms. Again they rise out of that, evolving for a certain period and slowly going back to the cause. So with all life. Each manifestation of life is coming up and then going back again. What goes down? The form. The form breaks to pieces, but it comes up again. In one sense bodies and forms even are eternal. How? Suppose we take a number of dice and throw them, and they fall in this ratio — 6 — 5 — 3 — 4. We take the dice up and throw them again and again; there must be a time when the same numbers will come again; the same combination must come. Now each particle, each atom, that is in this universe, I take for such a die, and these are being thrown out and combined again and again. All these forms before you are one combination. Here are the forms of a glass, a table, a pitcher of water, and so forth. This is one combination; in time, it will all break. But there must come a time when exactly the same combination comes again, when you will be here, and this form will be here, this subject will be talked, and this pitcher will be here. An infinite number of times this has been, and an infinite number of times this will be repeated. Thus far with the physical forms. What do we find? That even the combination of physical forms is eternally repeated.

A most interesting conclusion that follows from this theory is the explanation of facts such as these: Some of you, perhaps, have seen a man who can read the past life of others and foretell the future. How is it possible for any one to see what the future will be, unless there is a regulated future? Effects of the past will recur in the future, and we see that it is so. You have seen the big Ferris Wheel [1] in Chicago. The wheel revolves, and the little rooms in the wheel are regularly coming one after another; one set of persons gets into these, and after they have gone round the circle, they get out, and a fresh batch of people gets in. Each one of these batches is like one of these manifestations, from the lowest animals to the highest man. Nature is like the chain of the Ferris Wheel, endless and infinite, and these little carriages are the bodies or forms in which fresh batches of souls are riding, going up higher and higher until they become perfect and come out of the wheel. But the wheel goes on. And so long as the bodies are in the wheel, it can be absolutely and mathematically foretold where they will go, but not so of the souls. Thus it is possible to read the past and the future of nature with precision. We see, then, that there is recurrence of the same material phenomena at certain periods, and that the same combinations have been taking place through eternity. But that is not the immortality of the soul. No force can die, no matter can be annihilated. What becomes of it? It goes on changing, backwards and forwards, until it returns to the source from which it came. There is no motion in a straight line. Everything moves in a circle; a straight line, infinitely produced, becomes a circle. If that is the case, there cannot be eternal degeneration for any soul. It cannot be. Everything must complete the circle, and come back to its source. What are you and I and all these souls? In our discussion of evolution and involution, we have seen that you and I must be part of the cosmic consciousness, cosmic life, cosmic mind, which got involved and we must complete the circle and go back to this cosmic intelligence which is God. This cosmic intelligence is what people call Lord, or God, or Christ, or Buddha, or Brahman, what the materialists perceive as force, and the agnostics as that infinite, inexpressible beyond; and we are all parts of that.

This is the second idea, yet this is not sufficient; there will be still more doubts. It is very good to say that there is no destruction for any force. But all the forces and forms that we see are combinations. This form before us is a composition of several component parts, and so every force that we see is similarly composite. If you take the scientific idea of force, and call it the sum total, the resultant of several forces, what becomes of your individuality? Everything that is a compound must sooner or later go back to its component parts. Whatever in this universe is the result of the combination of matter or force must sooner or later go back to its components. Whatever is the result of certain causes must die, must be destroyed. It gets broken up, dispersed, and resolved back into its components. Soul is not a force; neither is it thought. It is the manufacturer of thought, but not thought itself; it is the manufacturer of the body, but not the body. Why so? We see that the body cannot be the soul. Why not? Because it is not intelligent. A corpse is not intelligent, nor a piece of meat in a butcher's shop. What do we mean by intelligence? Reactive power. We want to go a little more deeply into this. Here is a pitcher; I see it. How? Rays of light from the pitcher enter my eyes, and make a picture in my retina, which is carried to the brain. Yet there is no vision. What the physiologists call the sensory nerves carry this impression inwards. But up to this there is no reaction. The nerve centre in the brain carries the impression to the mind, and the mind reacts, and as soon as this reaction comes, the pitcher flashes before it. Take a more commonplace example. Suppose you are listening to me intently and a mosquito is sitting on the tip of your nose and giving you that pleasant sensation which mosquitoes can give; but you are so intent on hearing me that you do not feel the mosquito at all. What has happened? The mosquito has bitten a certain part of your skin, and certain nerves are there. They have carried a certain sensation to the brain, and the impression is there, but the mind, being otherwise occupied, does not react, so you are not aware of the presence of the mosquito. When a new impression comes, if the mind does not react, we shall not be conscious of it, but when the reaction comes we feel, we see, we hear, and so forth. With this reaction comes illumination, as the Sâmkhya philosophers call it. We see that the body cannot illuminate, because in the absence of attention no sensation is possible. Cases have been known where, under peculiar conditions, a man who had never learnt a particular language was found able to speak it. Subsequent inquiries proved that the man had, when a child, lived among people who spoke that language and the impressions were left in his brain. These impressions remained stored up there, until through some cause the mind reacted, and illumination came, and then the man was able to speak the language. This shows that the mind alone is not sufficient, that the mind itself is an instrument in the hands of someone. In the case of that boy the mind contained that language, yet he did not know it, but later there came a time when he did. It shows that there is someone besides the mind; and when the boy was a baby, that someone did not use the power; but when the boy grew up, he took advantage of it, and used it. First, here is the body, second the mind, or instrument of thought, and third behind this mind is the Self of man. The Sanskrit word is Atman. As modern philosophers have identified thought with molecular changes in the brain, they do not know how to explain such a case, and they generally deny it. The mind is intimately connected with the brain which dies every time the body changes. The Self is the illuminator, and the mind is the instrument in Its hands, and through that instrument It gets hold of the external instrument, and thus comes perception. The external instruments get hold of the impressions and carry them to the organs, for you must remember always, that the eyes and ears are only receivers — it is the internal organs, the brain centres, which act. In Sanskrit these centres are called Indriyas, and they carry sensations to the mind, and the mind presents them further back to another state of the mind, which in Sanskrit is called Chitta, and there they are organised into will, and all these present them to the King of kings inside, the Ruler on His throne, the Self of man. He then sees and gives His orders. Then the mind immediately acts on the organs, and the organs on the external body. The real Perceiver, the real Ruler, the Governor, the Creator, the Manipulator of all this, is the Self of man.

We see, then, that the Self of man is not the body, neither is It thought. It cannot be a compound. Why not? Because everything that is a compound can be seen or imagined. That which we cannot imagine or perceive, which we cannot bind together, is not force or matter, cause or effect, and cannot be a compound. The domain of compounds is only so far as our mental universe, our thought universe extends. Beyond this it does not hold good; it is as far as law reigns, and if there is anything beyond law, it cannot be a compound at all. The Self of man being beyond the law of causation, is not a compound. It is ever free and is the Ruler of everything that is within law. It will never die, because death means going back to the component parts, and that which was never a compound can never die. It is sheer nonsense to say It dies.

We are now treading on finer and finer ground, and some of you, perhaps, will be frightened. We have seen that this Self, being beyond the little universe of matter and force and thought, is a simple; and as a simple It cannot die. That which does not die cannot live. For life and death are the obverse and reverse of the same coin. Life is another name for death, and death for life. One particular mode of manifestation is what we call life; another particular mode of manifestation of the same thing is what we call death. When the wave rises on the top it is life; and when it falls into the hollow it is death. If anything is beyond death, we naturally see it must also be beyond life. I must remind you of the first conclusion that the soul of man is part of the cosmic energy that exists, which is God. We now find that it is beyond life and death. You were never born, and you will never die. What is this birth and death that we see around us? This belongs to the body only, because the soul is omnipresent. "How can that be?" you may ask. "So many people are sitting here, and you say the soul is omnipresent?" What is there, I ask, to limit anything that is beyond law, beyond causation? This glass is limited; it is not omnipresent, because the surrounding matter forces it to take that form, does not allow it to expand. It is conditioned be everything around it, and is, therefore, limited. But that which is beyond law, where there is nothing to act upon it, how can that be limited? It must be omnipresent. You are everywhere in the universe. How is it then that I am born and I am going to die, and all that? That is the talk of ignorance, hallucination of the brain. You were neither born, nor will you die. You have had neither birth, nor will have rebirth, nor life, nor incarnation, nor anything. What do you mean by coming and going? All shallow nonsense. You are everywhere. Then what is this coming and going? It is the hallucination produced by the change of this fine body which you call the mind. That is going on. Just a little speck of cloud passing before the sky. As it moves on and on, it may create the delusion that the sky moves. Sometimes you see a cloud moving before the moon, and you think that the moon is moving. When you are in a train you think the land is flying, or when you are in a boat, you think the water moves. In reality you are neither going nor coming, you are not being born, nor going to be reborn; you are infinite, ever-present, beyond all causation, and ever-free. Such a question is out of place, it is arrant nonsense. How could there be mortality when there was no birth?

One step more we will have to take to come to a logical conclusion. There is no half-way house. You are metaphysicians, and there is no crying quarter. If then we are beyond all law, we must be omniscient, ever-blessed; all knowledge must be in us and all power and blessedness. Certainly. You are the omniscient. Omnipresent being of the universe. But of such beings can there be many? Can there be a hundred thousand millions of omnipresent beings? Certainly not. Then, what becomes of us all? You are only one; there is only one such Self, and that One Self is you. Standing behind this little nature is what we call the Soul. There is only One Being, One Existence, the ever-blessed, the omnipresent, the omniscient, the birthless, deathless. "Through His control the sky expands, through His control the air breathes, through His control the sun shines, and through His control all live. He is the Reality in nature, He is the Soul of your soul, nay, more, you are He, you are one with Him." Wherever there are two, there is fear, there is danger, there is conflict, there is strife. When it is all One, who is there to hate, who is there to struggle with? When it is all He, with whom can you fight? This explains the true nature of life; this explains the true nature of being. This is perfection, and this is God. As long as you see the many, you are under delusion. "In this world of many he who sees the One, in this ever changing world he who sees Him who never changes, as the Soul of his own soul, as his own Self, he is free, he is blessed, he has reached the goal." Therefore know that thou art He; thou art the God of this universe, "Tat Tvam Asi" (That thou art). All these various ideas that I am a man or a woman, or sick or healthy, or strong or weak, or that I hate or I love, or have a little power, are but hallucinations. Away with them I What makes you weak? What makes you fear? You are the One Being in the universe. What frightens you? Stand up then and be free. Know that every thought and word that weakens you in this world is the only evil that exists. Whatever makes men weak and fear is the only evil that should be shunned. What can frighten you? If the suns come down, and the moons crumble into dust, and systems after systems are hurled into annihilation, what is that to you? Stand as a rock; you are indestructible. You are the Self, the God of the universe. Say – "I am Existence Absolute, Bliss Absolute, Knowledge Absolute, I am He," and like a lion breaking its cage, break your chain and be free for ever. What frightens you, what holds you down? Only ignorance and delusion; nothing else can bind you. You are the Pure One, the Ever-blessed.

Silly fools tell you that you are sinners, and you sit down in a corner and weep. It is foolishness, wickedness, downright rascality to say that you are sinners! You are all God. See you not God and call Him man? Therefore, if you dare, stand on that – mould your whole life on that. If a man cuts your throat, do not say no, for you are cutting your own throat. When you help a poor man, do not feel the least pride. That is worship for you, and not the cause of pride. Is not the whole universe you? Where is there any one that is not you? You are the Soul of this universe. You are the sun, moon, and stars, it is you that are shining everywhere. The whole universe is you. Whom are you going to hate or to fight? Know, then, that thou art He, and model your whole life accordingly; and he who knows this and models his life accordingly will no more grovel in darkness.

Notes

1. An amusement device consisting of a giant power-driven steel wheel, revolvable on its stationary axle, and carrying a number of balanced passenger cars around its rim."—Webster, G. W. G. Ferris erected the first of its kind for the Chicago Exposition of 1893. In India we have a corresponding wooden device very common in fairs. — Ed.

❑

14

The Atman

(*Delivered in America*)

Many of you have read Max Müller's celebrated book, *Three Lectures on the Vedanta Philosophy*, and some of you may, perhaps, have read, in German, Professor Deussen's book on the same philosophy. In what is being written and taught in the West about the religious thought of India, one school of Indian thought is principally represented, that which is called Advaitism, the monistic side of Indian religion; and sometimes it is thought that all the teachings of the Vedas are comprised in that one system of philosophy. There are, however, various phases of Indian thought; and, perhaps, this non-dualistic form is in the minority as compared with the other phases. From the most ancient times there have been various sects of thought in India, and as there never was a formulated or recognised church or any body of men to designate the doctrines which should be believed by each school, people were very free to choose their own form, make their own philosophy and establish their own sects. We, therefore, find that from the most ancient times India was full of religious sects. At the present time, I do not know how many hundreds of sects we have in India, and several fresh ones are coming into existence every year. It seems that the religious activity of that nation is simply inexhaustible.

Of these various sects, in the first place, there can be made two main divisions, the orthodox and the unorthodox. Those that believe in the Hindu scriptures, the Vedas, as eternal revelations of truth, are called orthodox, and those that stand on other authorities, rejecting the Vedas, are the heterodox in India. The chief modern unorthodox Hindu sects are the Jains and the Buddhists. Among the orthodox some declare that the scriptures are of much higher authority than reason; others again say that only that portion of the scriptures which is rational should be taken and the rest rejected.

Of the three orthodox divisions, the Sânkhyas, the Naiyâyikas, and the Mimâmsakas, the former two, although they existed as philosophical schools, failed to form any sect. The one sect that now really covers India is that of the later Mimamsakas or the Vedantists. Their philosophy is called Vedantism. All the schools of Hindu philosophy start from the Vedanta or Upanishads, but the monists took the name to themselves as a speciality, because they wanted to base the whole of their theology and philosophy upon the Vedanta and nothing else. In the course of time the Vedanta prevailed, and all the various sects of India that now exist can be referred to one or other of its schools. Yet these schools are not unanimous in their opinions.

We find that there are three principal variations among the Vedantists. On one point they all agree, and that is that they all believe in God. All these Vedantists also believe the Vedas to be the revealed word of God, not exactly in the same sense, perhaps, as the Christians or the Mohammedans believe, but in a very peculiar sense. Their idea is that the Vedas are an expression of the knowledge of God, and as God is eternal, His knowledge is eternally with Him, and so are the Vedas eternal. There is another common ground of belief: that of creation in cycles, that the whole of creation appears and disappears; that it is projected and becomes grosser and grosser, and at the end of an incalculable period of time it becomes finer and finer, when it dissolves and subsides, and then comes a period of rest. Again it: begins to appear and goes through the same process. They postulate the existence of a material which they call Âkâsha, which is something like the ether of the scientists, and a power which they call Prâna. About; this Prana they declare that by its vibration the universe is produced. When a cycle ends, all this manifestation of nature becomes finer and finer and dissolves into that Akasha which cannot be seen or felt, yet out of which everything is manufactured. All the forces that we see in nature, such as gravitation, attraction, and repulsion, or as thought, feeling, and nervous motion – all these various forces resolve into that Prana, and the vibration of the Prana ceases. In that state it remains until the beginning of the next cycle. Prana then begins to vibrate, and that vibration acts upon the Akasha, and all these forms are thrown out in regular succession.

The first school I will tell you about is styled the dualistic school. The dualists believe that God, who is the creator of the universe and its ruler, is eternally separate from nature, eternally separate from the human soul. God is eternal; nature is eternal; so are all souls. Nature and the souls become manifested and change, but God remains the same. According to the dualists, again, this God is personal in that He has qualities, not that He has a body. He has human attributes; He is merciful, He is just, He is powerful, He is almighty, He can be approached, He can be prayed to, He can be loved, He loves in return, and so forth. In one word, He is a human God, only infinitely greater than man; He has none of the evil qualities which men have. "He is the repository of an infinite number of blessed qualities" – that is their definition. He cannot create without materials, and nature is the material out of which He creates the whole universe. There are some non-Vedantic dualists, called "Atomists", who believe that nature is nothing but an infinite number of atoms, and God's will, acting upon these atoms, creates. The Vedantists deny the atomic theory; they say it is perfectly illogical. The indivisible atoms are like geometrical points without parts or magnitude; but something without parts or magnitude, if multiplied an infinite number of times, will remain the same. Anything that has no parts will never make something that has parts; any number of zeros added together will not make one single whole number. So, if these atoms are such that they have no parts or magnitude, the creation of the universe is simply impossible out of such atoms. Therefore, according to the Vedantic dualists, there is what they call indiscrete or undifferentiated nature, and out of that God creates the universe. The vast mass of Indian people are dualists. Human nature ordinarily cannot conceive of anything higher. We find that ninety per cent of the population of the earth who believe in any religion are dualists. All the religions of Europe and Western Asia are dualistic; they have to be. The ordinary man cannot think of anything which is not concrete. He naturally likes to cling to that which his intellect can grasp. That is to say, he can only conceive of higher spiritual ideas by bringing them down to his own level. He can only grasp abstract thoughts by making them concrete. This is the religion of the masses all over the world. They believe in a God who is entirely separate from them, a great king, a high, mighty monarch, as it were. At the same time they make Him purer than the monarchs of the earth; they give Him all good qualities and remove the evil qualities from Him. As if it were ever possible for good to exist without evil; as if there could be any conception of light without a conception of darkness!

With all dualistic theories the first difficulty is, how is it possible that under the rule of a just and merciful God, the repository of an infinite number of good qualities, there can be so many evils in this world? This question arose in all dualistic religions, but the Hindus never invented a Satan as an answer to it. The Hindus with one accord laid the blame on man, and it was easy for them to do so. Why? Because, as I have just now told you, they did not believe that souls were created out of nothing We see in this life that we can shape and form our future every one of us, every day, is trying to shape the morrow; today we fix the fate of the morrow; tomorrow we shall fix the fate of the day after, and so on. It is quite logical that this reasoning can be pushed backward too. If by our own deeds we shape our destiny in the future why not apply the same rule to the past? If, in an infinite chain, a certain number of links are alternately repeated then, if one of these groups of links be explained, we can explain the whole chain. So, in this infinite length of time, if we can cut off one portion and explain that portion and understand it, then, if it be true that nature is uniform, the same explanation must apply to the whole chain of time. If it be true that we are working out our own destiny here within this short space of time if it be true that everything must have a cause as we see it now, it must also be true that that which we are now is the effect of the whole of our past; therefore, no other person is necessary to shape the destiny of mankind but man himself. The evils that are in the world are caused by none else but ourselves. We have caused all this evil; and just as we constantly see misery resulting from evil actions, so can we also see that much of the existing misery in the world is the effect of the past wickedness of man. Man alone, therefore, according to this theory, is responsible. God is not to blame. He, the eternally merciful Father, is not to blame at all. "We reap what we sow."

Another peculiar doctrine of the dualists is, that every soul must eventually come to salvation. No one will be left out. Through various vicissitudes, through various sufferings and enjoyments, each one of them will come out in the end. Come out of what? The one common idea of all Hindu sects is that all souls have to get out of this universe. Neither the universe which we see and feel, nor even an imaginary one, can be right, the real one, because both are mixed up with good and evil. According to the dualists, there is beyond this universe a place full of happiness and good only; and when that place is reached, there will be no more necessity of being born and reborn, of living and dying; and this idea is very dear to them. No more disease there, and no more death. There will be eternal happiness, and they will be in the presence of God for all time and enjoy Him for ever. They believe that all beings, from the lowest worm up to the highest angels and gods, will all, sooner or later, attain to that world where there will be no more misery. But our world will never end; it goes on infinitely, although moving in waves. Although moving in cycles it never ends. The number of souls that are to be saved, that are to be perfected, is infinite. Some are in plants, some are in the lower animals, some are in men, some are in gods, but all of them, even the highest gods, are imperfect, are in bondage. What is the bondage? The necessity of being born and the necessity of dying. Even the highest gods die. What are these gods? They mean certain states, certain offices. For instance, Indra the king of gods, means a certain office; some soul which was very high has gone to fill that post in this cycle, and after this cycle he will be born again as man and come down to this earth, and the man who is very good in this cycle will go and fill that post in the next cycle. So with all these gods; they are certain offices which have been filled alternately by millions and millions of souls, who, after filling those offices, came down and became men. Those who do good works in this world and help others, but with an eye to reward, hoping to reach heaven or to get the praise of their fellow-men, must when they die, reap the benefit of those good works — they become these gods. But that is not salvation; salvation never will come through hope of reward. Whatever man desires the Lord gives him. Men desire power, they desire prestige, they desire enjoyments as gods, and they get these desires fulfilled, but no effect of work can be eternal. The effect will be exhausted after a certain length of time; it may be aeons, but after that it will be gone, and these gods must come down again and become men and get another chance for liberation. The lower animals will come up and become men, become gods, perhaps, then become men again, or go back to animals, until the time when they will get rid of all desire for enjoyment, the thirst for life, this clinging on to the "me and mine". This "me and mine" is the very root of all the evil in the world. If you ask a dualist, "Is your child yours?" he will say, "It is God's. My property is not mine, it is God's." Everything should be held as God's.

Now, these dualistic sects in India are great vegetarians, great preachers of non-killing of animals. But their idea about it is quite different from that of the Buddhist. If you ask a Buddhist, "Why do you preach against killing any animal?" he will answer, "We have no right to take any life;" and if you ask a dualist, "Why do you not kill any animal?" he says, "Because it is the Lord's." So the dualist says that this "me and mine" is to be applied to God and God alone; He is the only "me" and everything is His. When a man has come to the state when he has no "me and mine," when everything is given up to the Lord, when he loves everybody and is ready even to give up his life for an animal, without any desire for reward, then his heart will be purified, and when the heart has been purified, into that heart will come the love of God. God is the centre of attraction for every soul, and the dualist says, "A needle covered up with clay will not be attracted by a magnet, but as soon as the clay is washed off, it will be attracted." God is the magnet and human soul is the needle, and its evil works, the dirt and dust that cover it. As soon as the soul is pure it will by natural attraction come to God and remain with Him for ever, but remain eternally separate. The perfected soul, if it wishes, can take any form; it is able to take a hundred bodies, if it wishes or have none at all, if it so desires. It becomes almost almighty, except that it cannot create; that power belongs to God alone. None, however perfect, can manage the affairs of the universe; that function belongs to God. But all souls, when they become perfect, become happy for ever and live eternally with God. This is the dualistic statement.

One other idea the dualists preach. They protest against the idea of praying to God, "Lord, give me this and give me that." They think that should not be done. If a man must ask some material gift, he should ask inferior beings for it; ask one of these gods, or angels or a perfected being for temporal things. God is only to be loved. It is almost a blasphemy to pray to God, "Lord, give me this, and give me that." According to the dualists, therefore, what a man wants, he will get sooner or later, by praying to one of the gods; but if he wants salvation, he must worship God. This is the religion of the masses of India.

The real Vedanta philosophy begins with those known as the qualified non-dualists. They make the statement that the effect is never different from the cause; the effect is but the cause reproduced in another form. If the universe is the effect and God the cause, it must be God Himself – it cannot be anything but that. They start with the assertion that God is both the efficient and the material cause of the universe; that He Himself is the creator, and He Himself is the material out of which the whole of nature is projected. The word "creation" in your language has no equivalent in Sanskrit, because there is no sect in India which believes in creation, as it is regarded in the West, as something coming out of nothing. It seems that at one time there were a few that had some such idea, but they were very quickly silenced. At the present time I do not know of any sect that believes this. What we mean by creation is projection of that which already existed. Now, the whole universe, according to this sect, is God Himself. He is the material of the universe. We read in the Vedas, "As the Urnanâbhi (spider) spins the thread out of its own body, . . . even so the whole universe has come out of the Being."

If the effect is the cause reproduced, the question is: "How is it that we find this material, dull, unintelligent universe produced from a God, who is not material, but who is eternal intelligence? How, if the cause is pure and perfect, can the effect be quite different?" What do these qualified non-dualists say? Theirs is a very peculiar theory. They say that these three existences, God, nature, and the soul, are one. God is, as it were, the Soul, and nature and souls are the body of God. Just as I have a body and I have a soul, so the whole universe and all souls are the body of God, and God is the Soul of souls. Thus, God is the material cause of the universe. The body may be changed — may be young or old, strong or weak — but that does not affect the soul at all. It is the same eternal existence, manifesting through the body. Bodies come and go, but the soul does not change. Even so the whole universe is the body of God, and in that sense it is God. But the change in the universe does not affect God. Out of this material He creates the universe, and at the end of a cycle His body becomes finer, it contracts; at the beginning of another cycle it becomes expanded again, and out of it evolve all these different worlds.

Now both the dualists and the qualified non-dualists admit that the soul is by its nature pure, but through its own deeds it becomes impure. The qualified non-dualists express it more beautifully than the dualists, by saving that the soul's purity and perfection become contracted and again become manifest, and what we are now trying to do is to remanifest the intelligence, the purity, the power which is natural to the soul. Souls have a multitude of qualities, but not that of almightiness or all-knowingness. Every wicked deed contracts the nature of the soul, and every good deed expands it, and these souls, are all parts of

God. "As from a blazing fire fly millions of sparks of the same nature, even so from this Infinite Being, God, these souls have come." Each has the same goal. The God of the qualified non-dualists is also a Personal God, the repository of an infinite number of blessed qualities, only He is interpenetrating everything in the universe. He is immanent in everything and everywhere; and when the scriptures say that God is everything, it means that God is interpenetrating everything, not that God has become the wall, but that God is in the wall. There is not a particle, not an atom in the universe where He is not. Souls are all limited; they are not omnipresent. When they get expansion of their powers and become perfect, there is no more birth and death for them; they live with God for ever.

Now we come to Advaitism, the last and, what we think, the fairest flower of philosophy and religion that any country in any age has produced, where human thought attains its highest expression and even goes beyond the mystery which seems to be impenetrable. This is the non-dualistic Vedantism. It is too abstruse, too elevated to be the religion of the masses. Even in India, its birthplace, where it has been ruling supreme for the last three thousand years, it has not been able to permeate the masses. As we go on we shall find that it is difficult for even the most thoughtful man and woman in any country to understand Advaitism. We have made ourselves so weak; we have made ourselves so low. We may make great claims, but naturally we want to lean on somebody else. We are like little, weak plants, always wanting a support. How many times I have been asked for a "comfortable religion!" Very few men ask for the truth, fewer still dare to learn the truth, and fewest of all dare to follow it in all its practical bearings. It is not their fault; it is all weakness of the brain. Any new thought, especially of a high kind, creates a disturbance, tries to make a new channel, as it were, in the brain matter, and that unhinges the system, throws men off their balance. They are used to certain surroundings, and have to overcome a huge mass of ancient superstitions, ancestral superstition, class superstition, city superstition, country superstition, and behind all, the vast mass of superstition that is innate in every human being. Yet there are a few brave souls in the world who dare to conceive the truth, who dare to take it up, and who dare to follow it to the end.

What does the Advaitist declare? He says, if there is a God, that God must be both the material and the efficient cause of the universe. Not only is He the creator, but He is also the created. He Himself is this universe. How can that be? God, the pure, the spirit, has become the universe? Yes; apparently so. That which all ignorant people see as the universe does not really exist. What are you and I and all these things we see? Mere self-hypnotism; there is but one Existence, the Infinite, the Ever-blessed One. In that Existence we dream all these various dreams. It is the Atman, beyond all, the Infinite, beyond the known, beyond the knowable; in and through That we see the universe. It is the only Reality. It is this table; It is the audience before me; It is the wall; It is everything, minus the name and form. Take away the form of the table, take away the name; what remains is It. The Vedantist does not call It either He or She — these are fictions, delusions of the human brain — there is no sex in the soul. People who are under illusion, who have become like animals, see a woman or a man; living gods do not see men or women. How can they who are beyond everything have any sex idea? Everyone and everything is the Atman — the Self — the sexless, the pure, the ever-blessed. It is the name, the form, the body, which are material, and they make all this difference. If you take away these two differences of name and form, the whole universe is one; there are no two, but one everywhere. You and I are one. There is neither nature, nor God, nor the universe, only that one Infinite Existence, out of which, through name and form, all these are manufactured. How to know the Knower? It cannot be known. How can you see your own Self? You can only reflect yourself. So all this universe is the reflection of that One Eternal Being, the Atman, and as the reflection falls upon good or bad reflectors, so good or bad images are cast up. Thus in the murderer, the reflector is bad and not the Self. In the saint the reflector is pure. The Self — the Atman

— is by Its own nature pure. It is the same, the one Existence of the universe that is reflecting Itself from the lowest worm to the highest and most perfect being. The whole of this universe is one Unity, one Existence, physically, mentally, morally and spiritually. We are looking upon this one Existence in different forms and creating all these images upon It. To the being who has limited himself to the condition of man, It appears as the world of man. To the being who is on a higher plane of existence, It may seem like heaven. There is but one Soul in the universe, not two. It neither comes nor goes. It is neither born, nor dies, nor reincarnates. How can It die? Where can It go? All these heavens, all these earths, and all these places are vain imaginations of the mind. They do not exist, never existed in the past, and never will exist in the future.

I am omnipresent, eternal. Where can I go? Where am I not already? I am reading this book of nature. Page after page I am finishing and turning over, and one dream of life after another goes Away. Another page of life is turned over; another dream of life comes, and it goes away, rolling and rolling, and when I have finished my reading, I let it go and stand aside, I throw away the book, and the whole thing is finished. What does the Advaitist preach? He dethrones all the gods that ever existed, or ever will exist in the universe and places on that throne the Self of man, the Atman, higher than the sun and the moon, higher than the heavens, greater than this great universe itself. No books, no scriptures, no science can ever imagine the glory of the Self that appears as man, the most glorious God that ever was, the only God that ever existed, exists, or ever will exist. I am to worship, therefore, none but myself. "I worship my Self," says the Advaitist. To whom shall I bow down? I salute my Self. To whom shall I go for help? Who can help me, the Infinite Being of the universe? These are foolish dreams, hallucinations; who ever helped any one? None. Wherever you see a weak man, a dualist, weeping and wailing for help from somewhere above the skies, it is because he does not know that the skies also are in him. He wants help from the skies, and the help comes. We see that it comes; but it comes from within himself, and he mistakes it as coming from without. Sometimes a sick man lying on his bed may hear a tap on the door. He gets up and opens it and finds no one there. He goes back to bed, and again he hears a tap. He gets up and opens the door. Nobody is there. At last he finds that it was his own heartbeat which he fancied was a knock at the door. Thus man, after this vain search after various gods outside himself, completes the circle, and comes back to the point from which he started – the human soul, and he finds that the God whom he was searching in hill and dale, whom he was seeking in every brook, in every temple, in churches and heavens, that God whom he was even imagining as sitting in heaven and ruling the world, is his own Self. I am He, and He is I. None but I was God, and this little I never existed.

Yet, how could that perfect God have been deluded? He never was. How could a perfect God have been dreaming? He never dreamed. Truth never dreams. The very question as to whence this illusion arose is absurd. Illusion arises from illusion alone. There will be no illusion as soon as the truth is seen. Illusion always rests upon illusion; it never rests upon God, the Truth, the Atman. You are never in illusion; it is illusion that is in you, before you. A cloud is here; another comes and pushes it aside and takes its place. Still another comes and pushes that one away. As before the eternal blue sky, clouds of various hue and colour come, remain for a short time and disappear, leaving it the same eternal blue, even so are you, eternally pure, eternally perfect. You are the veritable Gods of the universe; nay, there are not two – there is but One. It is a mistake to say, "you and I"; say "I". It is I who am eating in millions of mouths; how can I be hungry? It is I who am working through an infinite number of hands; how can I be inactive? It is I who am living the life of the whole universe; where is death for me? I am beyond all life, beyond all death. Where shall I seek for freedom? I am free by my nature. Who can bind me – the God of this universe? The scriptures of the world are but little maps, wanting to delineate my glory, who am the only existence of the universe. Then what are these books to me? Thus says the Advaitist.

"Know the truth and be free in a moment." All the darkness will then vanish. When man has seen himself as one with the Infinite Being of the universe, when all separateness has ceased, when all men and women, an gods and angels, all animals and plants, and the whole universe have melted into that Oneness, then all fear disappears. Can I hurt myself? Can I kill myself? Can I injure myself? Whom to fear? Can you fear yourself? Then will all sorrow disappear. What can cause me sorrow? I am the One Existence of the universe. Then all jealousies will disappear; of whom to be jealous? Of myself? Then all bad feelings disappear. Against whom can I have bad feeling? Against myself? There is none in the universe but I. And this is the one way, says the Vedantist, to Knowledge. Kill out this differentiation, kill out this superstition that there are many. "He who in this world of many sees that One, he who in this mass of insentiency sees that one Sentient Being, he who in this world of shadows catches that Reality, unto him belongs eternal peace, unto none else, unto none else."

These are the salient points of the three steps which Indian religious thought has taken in regard to God. We have seen that it began with the Personal, the extra-cosmic God. It went from the external to the internal cosmic body, God immanent in the universe, and ended in identifying the soul itself with that God, and making one Soul, a unit of all these various manifestations in the universe. This is the last word of the Vedas. It begins with dualism, goes through a qualified monism and ends in perfect monism. We know how very few in this world can come to the last, or even dare believe in it, and fewer still dare act according to it. Yet we know that therein lies the explanation of all ethics, of all morality and all spirituality in the universe. Why is it that every one says, "Do good to others?" Where is the explanation? Why is it that all great men have preached the brotherhood of mankind, and greater men the brotherhood of all lives? Because whether they were conscious of it or not, behind all that, through all their irrational and personal superstitions, was peering forth the eternal light of the Self denying all manifoldness, and asserting that the whole universe is but one.

Again, the last word gave us one universe, which through the senses we see as matter, through the intellect as souls, and through the spirit as God. To the man who throws upon himself veils, which the world calls wickedness and evil, this very universe will change and become a hideous place; to another man, who wants enjoyments, this very universe will change its appearance and become a heaven, and to the perfect man the whole thing will vanish and become his own Self.

Now, as society exists at the present time, all these three stages are necessary; the one does not deny the other, one is simply the fulfilment of the other. The Advaitist or the qualified Advaitist does not say that dualism is wrong; it is a right view, but a lower one. It is on the way to truth; therefore let everybody work out his own vision of this universe, according to his own ideas. Injure none, deny the position of none; take man where he stands and, if you can, lend him a helping hand and put him on a higher platform, but do not injure and do not destroy. All will come to truth in the long run. "When all the desires of the heart will be vanquished, then this very mortal will become immortal" – then the very man will become God.

❑

15

The Atman: Its Bondage and Freedom

(*Delivered in America*)

According to the Advaita philosophy, there is only one thing real in the universe, which it calls Brahman; everything else is unreal, manifested and manufactured out of Brahman by the power of Mâyâ. To reach back to that Brahman is our goal. We are, each one of us, that Brahman, that Reality, plus this Maya. If we can get rid of this Maya or ignorance, then we become what we really are. According to this philosophy, each man consists of three parts – the body, the internal organ or the mind, and behind that, what is called the Âtman, the Self. The body is the external coating and the mind is the internal coating of the Atman who is the real perceiver, the real enjoyer, the being in the body who is working the body by means of the internal organ or the mind.

The Âtman is the only existence in the human body which is immaterial. Because it is immaterial, it cannot be a compound, and because it is not a compound, it does not obey the law of cause and effect, and so it is immortal. That which is immortal can have no beginning because everything with a beginning must have an end. It also follows that it must be formless; there cannot be any form without matter. Everything that has form must have a beginning and an end. We have none of us seen a form which had not a beginning and will not have an end. A form comes out of a combination of force and matter. This chair has a peculiar form, that is to say a certain quantity of matter is acted upon by a certain amount of force and made to assume a particular shape. The shape is the result of a combination of matter and force. The combination cannot be eternal; there must come to every combination a time when it will dissolve. So all forms have a beginning and an end. We know our body will perish; it had a beginning and it will have an end. But the Self having no form, cannot be bound by the law of beginning and end. It is existing from infinite time; just as time is eternal, so is the Self of man eternal. Secondly, it must be all-pervading. It is only form that is conditioned and limited by space; that which is formless cannot be confined in space. So, according to Advaita Vedanta, the Self, the Atman, in you, in me, in every one, is omnipresent. You are as much in the sun now as in this earth, as much in England as in America. But the Self acts through the mind and the body, and where they are, its action is visible.

Each work we do, each thought we think, produces an impression, called in Sanskrit Samskâra, upon the mind and the sum total of these impressions becomes the tremendous force which is called "character". The character of a man is what he has created for himself; it is the result of the mental and physical actions that he has done in his life. The sum total of the Samskaras is the force which gives a man the next direction after death. A man dies; the body falls away and goes back to the elements; but the Samskaras remain, adhering to the mind which, being made of fine material, does not dissolve, because the finer the material, the more persistent it is. But the mind also dissolves in the long run, and that is what we are struggling for. In this connection, the best illustration that comes to my mind is that of the whirlwind. Different currents of air coming from different directions meet and at the meeting-point become united and go on rotating; as they rotate, they form a body of dust, drawing in bits of paper, straw, etc., at one place, only to drop them and go on to another, and so go on rotating, raising and forming bodies out of the materials which are before them. Even so the forces, called Prâna in Sanskrit, come together and form the body and the mind out of matter, and move on until the body falls down, when they raise other materials to make another body, and when this falls, another rises, and thus the process goes on. Force cannot travel without matter. So when the body falls down, the mind-stuff remains, Prana in the form of Samskaras acting on it; and then it goes on to another point, raises up another whirl from fresh materials, and begins another motion; and so it travels from place to place until the force is all spent; and then it falls down, ended. So when the mind will end, be broken to pieces entirely, without leaving any Samskara, we shall be entirely free, and until that time we are in bondage; until then the Atman is covered by the whirl of the mind, and imagines it is being taken from place to place. When the whirl falls down, the Atman finds that It is all-pervading. It can go where It likes, is entirely free, and is able to manufacture any number of minds or bodies It likes; but until then It can go only with the whirl. This freedom is the goal towards which we are all moving.

Suppose there is a ball in this room, and we each have a mallet in our hands and begin to strike the ball, giving it hundreds of blows, driving it from point to point, until at last it flies out of the room. With what force and in what direction will it go out? These will be determined by the forces that have been acting upon it all through the room. All the different blows that have been given will have their effects. Each one of our actions, mental and physical, is such a blow. The human mind is a ball which is being hit. We are being hit about this room of the world all the time, and our passage out of it is determined by the force of all these blows. In each case, the speed and direction of the ball is determined by the hits it has received; so all our actions in this world will determine our future birth. Our present birth, therefore, is the result of our past. This is one case: suppose I give you an endless chain, in which there is a black link and a white link alternately, without beginning and without end, and suppose I ask you the nature of the chain. At first you will find a difficulty in determining its nature, the chain being infinite at both ends, but slowly you find out it is a chain. You soon discover that this infinite chain is a repetition of the two links, black and white, and these multiplied infinitely become a whole chain. If you know the nature of one of these links, you know the nature of the whole chain, because it is a perfect repetition. All our lives, past, present, and future, form, as it were, an infinite chain, without beginning and without end, each link of which is one life, with two ends, birth and death. What we are and do here is being repeated again and again, with but little variation. So if we know these two links, we shall know all the passages we shall have to pass through in this world. We see, therefore, that our passage into this world has been exactly determined by our previous passages. Similarly we are in this world by our own actions. Just as we go out with the sum total of our present actions upon us, so we see that we come into it with the sum total of our past actions upon us; that which takes us out is the very same thing that brings us in. What brings us in? Our past deeds. What takes us out? Our own deeds *here*, and so on and on we go. Like the caterpillar that takes the thread from its own mouth and builds its cocoon and at last finds itself caught inside the cocoon, we have bound ourselves by our own actions, we have thrown the network of our actions around ourselves. We have set the law of causation in motion, and we find it hard to get ourselves out of it. We have set the wheel in motion, and we are being crushed under it. So this philosophy teaches us that we are uniformly being bound by our own actions, good or bad.

The Atman never comes nor goes, is never born nor dies. It is nature moving before the Atman, and the reflection of this motion is on the Atman; and the Atman ignorantly thinks it is moving, and not nature. When the Atman thinks that, it is in bondage; but when it comes to find it never moves, that it is omnipresent, then freedom comes. The Atman in bondage is called Jiva. Thus you see that when it is said that the Atman comes and goes, it is said only for facility of understanding, just as for convenience in studying astronomy you are asked to suppose that the sun moves round the earth, though such is not the case. So the Jiva, the soul, comes to higher or lower states. This is the well-known law of reincarnation; and this law binds all creation.

People in this country think it too horrible that man should come up from an animal. Why? What will be the end of these millions of animals? Are they nothing? If we have a soul, so have they, and if they have none, neither have we. It is absurd to say that man alone has a soul, and the animals none. I have seen men worse than animals.

The human soul has sojourned in lower and higher forms, migrating from one to another, according to the Samskaras or impressions, but it is only in the highest form as man that it attains to freedom. The man form is higher than even the angel form, and of all forms it is the highest; man is the highest being in creation, because he attains to freedom.

All this universe was in Brahman, and it was, as it were, projected out of Him, and has been moving on to go back to the source from which it was projected, like the electricity which comes out of the dynamo, completes the circuit, and returns to it. The same is the case with the soul. Projected from Brahman, it passed through all sorts of vegetable and animal forms, and at last it is in man, and man is the nearest approach to Brahman. To go back to Brahman from which we have been projected is the great struggle of life. Whether people know it or not does not matter. In the universe, whatever we see of motion, of struggles in minerals or plants or animals is an effort to come back to the centre and be at rest. There was an equilibrium, and that has been destroyed; and all parts and atoms and molecules are struggling to find their lost equilibrium again. In this struggle they are combining and re-forming, giving rise to all the wonderful phenomena of nature. All struggles and competitions in animal life, plant life, and everywhere else, all social struggles and wars are but expressions of that eternal struggle to get back to that equilibrium.

The going from birth to death, this travelling, is what is called Samsara in Sanskrit, the round of birth and death literally. All creation, passing through this round, will sooner or later become free. The question may be raised that if we all shall come to freedom, why should we *struggle* to attain it? If every one is going to be free, we will sit down and wait. It is true that every being will become free, sooner or later; no one can be lost. Nothing can come to destruction; everything must come up. If that is so, what is the use of our struggling? In the first place, the struggle is the only means that will bring us to the centre, and in the second place, we do not know why we struggle. We have to. "Of thousands of men some are awakened to the idea that they will become free." The vast masses of mankind are content with material things, but there are some who awake, and want to get back, who have had enough of this playing, down here. These struggle consciously, while the rest do it unconsciously.

The alpha and omega of Vedanta philosophy is to "give up the world," giving up the unreal and taking the real. Those who are enamoured of the world may ask, "Why should we attempt to get out of it, to go back to the centre? Suppose we have all come from God, but we find this world is pleasurable and nice; then why should we not rather try to get more and more of the world? Why should we try to get out of it?" They say, look at the wonderful improvements going on in the world every day, how much luxury is being manufactured for it. This is very enjoyable. Why should we go away, and strive for something which is not this? The answer is that the world is certain to die, to be broken into pieces and that many times we have had the same enjoyments. All the forms which we are seeing now have been manifested again and again, and the world in which we live has been here many times before. I have been here and talked to you many times before. You will know that it must be so, and the very words that you have been listening to now, you have heard many times before. And many times more it will be the same. Souls were never different, the bodies have been constantly dissolving and recurring. Secondly, these things periodically occur. Suppose here are three or four dice, and when we throw them, one comes up five, another four, another three, and another two. If you keep on throwing, there must come times when those very same numbers will recur. Go on throwing, and no matter how long may be the interval, those numbers must come again. It cannot be asserted in how many throws they will come again; this is the law of chance. So with souls and their associations. However distant may be the periods, the same combinations and dissolutions will happen again and again. The same birth, eating and drinking, and then death, come round again and again. Some never find anything higher than the enjoyments of the world, but those who want to soar higher find that these enjoyments are never final, are only by the way.

Every form, let us say, beginning from the little worm and ending in man, is like one of the cars of the Chicago Ferris Wheel which is in motion all the time, but the occupants change. A man goes into a car, moves with the wheel, and comes out. The wheel goes on and on. A soul enters one form, resides in it for a time, then leaves it and goes into another and quits that again for a third. Thus the round goes on till it comes out of the wheel and becomes free.

Astonishing powers of reading the past and the future of a man's life have been known in every country and every age. The explanation is that so long as the Atman is within the realm of causation – though its inherent freedom is not entirely lost and can assert itself, even to the extent of taking the soul out of the causal chain, as it does in the case of men who become free – its actions are greatly influenced by the causal law and thus make it possible for men, possessed with the insight to trace the sequence of effects, to tell the past and the future.

So long as there is desire or want, it is a sure sign that there is imperfection. A perfect, free being cannot have any desire. God cannot want anything. If He desires, He cannot be God. He will be imperfect. So all the talk about God desiring this and that, and becoming angry and pleased by turns is babies' talk, but means nothing. Therefore it has been taught by all teachers, "Desire nothing, give up all desires and be perfectly satisfied."

A child comes into the world crawling and without teeth, and the old man gets out without teeth and crawling. The extremes are alike, but the one has no experience of the life before him, while the other has gone through it all. When the vibrations of ether are very low, we do not see light, it is darkness; when very high, the result is also darkness. The extremes generally appear to be the same, though one is as distant from the other as the poles. The wall has no desires, so neither has the perfect man. But the wall is not sentient enough to desire, while for the perfect man there is nothing to desire. There are idiots who have no desires in this world, because their brain is imperfect. At the same time, the highest state is when we have no desires, but the two are opposite poles of the same existence. One is near the animal, and the other near to God.

❑

16

The Real and the Apparent Man

(*Delivered in New York*)

Here we stand, and our eyes look forward sometimes miles ahead. Man has been doing that since he began to think. He is always looking forward, looking ahead. He wants to know where he goes even after the dissolution of his body. Various theories have been propounded, system after system has been brought forward to suggest explanations. Some have been rejected, while others have been accepted, and thus it will go on, so long as man is here, so long as man thinks. There is some truth in each of these systems. There is a good deal of what is not truth in all of them. I shall try to place before you the sum and substance, the result, of the inquiries in this line that have been made in India. I shall try to harmonise the various thoughts on the subject, as they have come up from time to time among Indian philosophers. I shall try to harmonise the psychologists and the metaphysicians, and, if possible, I shall harmonise them with modern scientific thinkers also.

The one theme of the Vedanta philosophy is the search after unity. The Hindu mind does not care for the particular; it is always after the general, nay, the universal. "What is that, by knowing which everything else is to be known?" That is the one theme. "As through the knowledge of one lump of clay all that is of clay is known, so, what is that, by knowing which this whole universe itself will be known?" That is the one search. The whole of this universe, according to the Hindu philosophers, can be resolved into one material, which they call Âkâsha. Everything that we see around us, feel, touch, taste, is simply a differentiated manifestation of this Akasha. It is all-pervading, fine. All that we call solids, liquids, or gases, figures, forms, or bodies, the earth, sun, moon, and stars – everything is composed of this Akasha.

What force is it which acts upon this Akasha and manufactures this universe out of it? Along with Akasha exists universal power; all that is power in the universe, manifesting as force or attraction – nay, even as thought – is but a different manifestation of that one power which the Hindus call Prâna. This Prana, acting on Akasha, is creating the whole of this universe. In the beginning of a cycle, this Prana, as it were, sleeps in the infinite ocean of Akasha. It existed motionless in the beginning. Then arises motion in this ocean of Akasha by the action of this Prana, and as this Prana begins to move, to vibrate, out of this ocean come the various celestial systems, suns, moons, stars, earth, human beings, animals, plants, and the manifestations of all the various forces and phenomena. Every manifestation of power, therefore, according to them, is this Prana. Every material manifestation is Akasha. When this cycle will end, all that we call solid will melt away into the next form, the next finer or the liquid form; that will melt into the gaseous, and that into finer and more uniform heat vibrations, and all will melt back into the original Akasha, and what we now call attraction, repulsion, and motion, will slowly resolve into the original Prana. Then this Prana is said to sleep for a period, again to emerge and to throw out all those forms; and when this period will end, the whole thing will subside again. Thus this process of creation is going down, and coming up, oscillating backwards and forwards. In the language of modern science, it is becoming static during one period, and during another period it is becoming dynamic. At one time it becomes potential, and at the next period it becomes active. This alteration has gone on through eternity.

Yet, this analysis is only partial. This much has been known even to modern physical science. Beyond that, the research of physical science cannot reach. But the inquiry does not stop in consequence. We have not yet found that one, by knowing which everything else will be known. We have resolved the whole universe into two components, into what are called matter and energy, or what the ancient philosophers of India called Akasha and Prana. The next step is to resolve this Akasha and the Prana into their origin. Both can be resolved into the still higher entity which is called mind. It is out of mind, the Mahat, the universally existing thought-power, that these two have been produced. Thought is a still finer manifestation of being than either Akasha or Prana. It is thought that splits itself into these two. The universal thought existed in the beginning, and that manifested, changed, evolved itself into these two Akasha and Prana: and by the combination of these two the whole universe has been produced.

We next come to psychology. I am looking at you. The external sensations are brought to me by the eyes; they are carried by the sensory nerves to the brain. The eyes are not the organs of vision. They are but the external instruments, because if the real organ behind, that which carries the sensation to the brain, is destroyed, I may have twenty eyes, yet I cannot see you. The picture on the retina may be as complete as possible, yet I shall not see you. Therefore, the organ is different from its instruments; behind the instruments, the eyes, there must be the organ So it is with all the sensations. The nose is not the sense of smell; it is but the instrument, and behind it is the organ. With every sense we have, there is first the external instrument in the physical body; behind that in the same physical body, there is the organ; yet these are not sufficient. Suppose I am talking to you, and you are listening to me with close attention. Something happens, say, a bell rings; you will not, perhaps, hear the bell ring. The pulsations of that sound came to your ear, struck the tympanum, the impression was carried by the nerve into the brain; if the whole process was complete up to carrying the impulse to the brain, why did you not hear? Something else was wanting – the mind was not attached to the organ. When the mind detaches itself from the organ, the organ may bring any news to it, but the mind will not receive it. When it attaches itself to the organ, then alone is it possible for the mind to receive the news. Yet, even that does not complete the whole. The instruments may bring the sensation from outside, the organs may carry it inside, the mind may attach itself to the organ, and yet the perception may not be complete. One more factor is necessary; there must be a reaction within. With this reaction comes knowledge. That which is outside sends, as it were, the current of news into my brain. My mind takes it up, and presents it to the intellect, which groups it in relation to pre-received impressions and sends a current of reaction, and with that reaction comes perception. Here, then, is the will. The state of mind which reacts is called Buddhi, the intellect. Yet, even this does not complete the whole. One step more is required. Suppose here is a camera and there is a sheet of cloth, and I try to throw a picture on that sheet. What am I to do? I am to guide various rays of light through the camera to fall upon the sheet and become grouped there. Something is necessary to have the picture thrown upon, which does not move. I cannot form a picture upon something which is moving; that something must be stationary, because the rays of light which I throw on it are moving, and these moving rays of light, must be gathered, unified, co-ordinated, and completed upon something which is stationary. Similar is the case with the sensations which these organs of ours are carrying inside and presenting to the mind, and which the mind in its turn is presenting to the intellect. This process will not be complete unless there is something permanent in the background upon which the picture, as it were, may be formed, upon which we may unify all the different impressions. What is it that gives unity to the changing whole of our being? What is it that keeps up the identity of the moving thing moment after moment? What is it upon which all our different impressions are pieced together, upon which the perceptions, as it were, come together, reside, and form a united whole? We have found that to serve this end there must be something, and we also see that that something must be, relatively to the body and mind, motionless. The sheet of cloth upon which the camera throws the picture is, relatively to the rays of light, motionless, else there will be no picture. That is to say, the perceiver must be an individual. This something upon which the mind is painting all these pictures, this something upon which our sensations, carried by the mind and intellect, are placed and grouped and formed into a unity, is what is called the soul of man.

We have seen that it is the universal cosmic mind that splits itself into the Akasha and Prana, and beyond mind we have found the soul in us. In the universe, behind the universal mind, there is a Soul that exists, and it is called God. In the individual it is the soul of man. In this universe, in the cosmos, just as the universal mind becomes evolved into Akasha and Prana, even so, we may find that the Universal Soul Itself becomes evolved as mind. Is it really so with the individual man? Is his mind the creator of his body, and his soul the creator of his mind? That is to say, are his body, his mind, and his soul three different existences or are they three in one or, again, are they different states of existence of the same unit being? We shall gradually try to find an answer to this question. The first step that we have now gained is this: here is this external body, behind this external body are the organs, the mind, the intellect, and behind this is the soul. At the first step, we have found, as it were, that the soul is separate from the body, separate from the mind itself. Opinions in the religious world become divided at this point, and the departure is this. All those religious views which generally pass under the name of dualism hold that this soul is qualified, that it is of various qualities, that all feelings of enjoyment, pleasure, and pain really belong to the soul. The non-dualists deny that the soul has any such qualities; they say it is unqualified.

Let me first take up the dualists, and try to present to you their position with regard to the soul and its destiny; next, the system that contradicts them; and lastly, let us try to find the harmony which non-dualism will bring to us. This soul of man, because it is separate from the mind and body, because it is not composed of Akasha and Prana, must be immortal. Why? What do we mean by mortality? Decomposition. And that is only possible for things that are the result of composition; anything that is made of two or three ingredients must become decomposed. That alone which is not the result of composition can never become decomposed, and, therefore, can never die. It is immortal. It has been existing throughout eternity; it is uncreate. Every item of creation is simply a composition; no one ever saw creation come out of nothing. All that we know of creation is the combination of already existing things into newer forms. That being so, this soul of man, being simple, must have been existing for ever, and it will exist for ever. When this body falls off, the soul lives on. According to the Vedantists, when this body dissolves, the vital forces of the man go back to his mind and the mind becomes dissolved, as it were, into the Prana, and that Prana enters into the soul of man, and the soul of man comes out, clothed, as it were, with what they call the fine body, the mental body, or spiritual body, as you may like to call it. In this body are the Samskâras of the man. What are the Samskaras? This mind is like a lake, and every thought is like a wave upon that lake. Just as in the lake waves rise and then fall down and disappear, so these thought-waves are continually rising in the mind-stuff and then disappearing, but they do not disappear for ever. They become finer and finer, but they are all there, ready to start up at another time when called upon to do so. Memory is simply calling back into waveform some of those thoughts which have gone into that finer state of existence. Thus, everything that we have thought, every action that we have done, is lodged in the mind; it is all there in fine form, and when a man dies, the sum total of these impressions is in the mind, which again works upon a little fine material as a medium. The soul, clothed, as it were, with these impressions and the fine body, passes out, and the destiny of the soul is guided by the resultant of all the different forces represented by the different impressions. According to us, there are three different goals for the soul.

Those that are very spiritual, when they die, follow the solar rays and reach what is called the solar sphere, through which they reach what is called the lunar sphere, and through that they reach what is called the sphere of lightning, and there they meet with another soul who is already blessed, and he guides the new-comer forward to the highest of all spheres, which is called the Brahmaloka, the sphere of Brahmâ. There these souls attain to omniscience and omnipotence, become almost as powerful and all-knowing as God Himself; and they reside there for ever, according to the dualists, or, according to the non-dualists, they become one with the Universal at the end of the cycle. The next class of persons, who have been doing good work with selfish motives, are carried by the results of their good works, when they die, to what is called lunar sphere, where there are various heavens, and there they acquire fine bodies, the bodies of gods. They become gods and live there and enjoy the blessing of heaven for a long period; and after that period is finished, the old Karma is again upon them, and so they fall back again to the earth; they come down through the spheres of air and clouds and all these various regions, and, at last, reach the earth through raindrops. There on the earth they attach themselves to some cereal which is eventually eaten by some man who is fit to supply them with material to make a new body. The last class, namely, the wicked, when they die, become ghosts or demons, and live somewhere midway between the lunar sphere and this earth. Some try to disturb mankind, some are friendly; and after living there for some time they also fall back to the earth and become animals. After living for some time in an animal body they get released, and come back, and become men again, and thus get one more chance to work out their salvation. We see, then, that those who have nearly attained to perfection, in whom only very little of impurity remains, go to the Brahmaloka through the rays of the sun; those who were a middling sort of people, who did some good work here with the idea of going to heaven, go to the heavens in the lunar sphere and there obtain god-bodies; but they have again to become men and so have one more chance to become perfect. Those that are very wicked become ghosts and demons, and then they may have to become animals; after that they become men again and get another chance to perfect themselves. This earth is called the Karma-Bhumi, the sphere of Karma. Here alone man makes his good or bad Karma. When a man wants to go to heaven and does good works for that purpose, he becomes as good and does not as such store up any bad Karma. He just enjoys the effects of the good work he did on earth; and when this good Karma is exhausted, there come, upon him the resultant force of all the evil Karma he had previously stored up in life, and that brings him down again to this earth.

In the same way, those that become ghosts remain in that state, not giving rise to fresh Karma, but suffer the evil results of their past misdeeds, and later on remain for a time in an animal body without causing any fresh Karma. When that period is finished, they too become men again. The states of reward and punishment due to good and bad Karmas are devoid of the force generating fresh Karmas; they have only to be enjoyed or suffered. If there is an extraordinarily good or an extraordinarily evil Karma, it bears fruit very quickly. For instance, if a man has been doing many evil things all his life, but does one good act, the result of that good act will immediately appear, but when that result has been gone through, all the evil acts must produce their results also. All men who do certain good and great acts, but the general tenor of whose lives has not been correct, will become gods; and after living for some time in god-bodies, enjoying the powers of gods, they will have again to become men; when the power of the good acts is thus finished, the old evil comes up to be worked out. Those who do extraordinarily evil acts have to put on ghost and devil bodies, and when the effect of those evil actions is exhausted, the little good action which remains associated with them, makes them again become men. The way to Brahmaloka, from which there is no more fall or return, is called the Devayâna, i.e. the way to God; the way to heaven is known as Pitriyâna, i.e. the way to the fathers.

Man, therefore, according to the Vedanta philosophy, is the greatest being that is in the universe, and this world of work the best place in it, because only herein is the greatest and the best chance for him to become perfect. Angels or gods, whatever you may call them, have all to become men, if they want to become perfect. This is the great centre, the wonderful poise, and the wonderful opportunity — this human life.

We come next to the other aspect of philosophy. There are Buddhists who deny the whole theory of the soul that I have just now been propounding. "What use is there," says the Buddhist, "to assume something as the substratum, as the background of this body and mind? Why may we not allow thoughts to run on? Why admit a third substance beyond this organism, composed of mind and body, a third substance called the soul? What is its use? Is not this organism sufficient to explain itself? Why take anew a third something?" These arguments are very powerful. This reasoning is very strong. So far as outside research goes, we see that this organism is a sufficient explanation of itself — at least, many of us see it in that light. Why then need there be a soul as substratum, as a something which is neither mind nor body but stands as a background for both mind and body? Let there be only mind and body. Body is the name of a stream of matter continuously changing. Mind is the name of a stream of consciousness or thought continuously changing. What produces the apparent unity between these two? This unity does not really exist, let us say. Take, for instance, a lighted torch, and whirl it rapidly before you. You see a circle of fire. The circle does not really exist, but because the torch is continually moving, it leaves the appearance of a circle. So there is no unity in this life; it is a mass of matter continually rushing down, and the whole of this matter you may call one unity, but no more. So is mind; each thought is separate from every other thought; it is only the rushing current that leaves behind the illusion of unity; there is no need of a third substance. This universal phenomenon of body and mind is all that really is; do not posit something behind it. You will find that this Buddhist thought has been taken up by certain sects and schools in modern times, and all of them claim that it is new — their own invention. This has been the central idea of most of the Buddhistic philosophies, that this world is itself all-sufficient; that you need not ask for any background at all; all that is, is this sense-universe: what is the use of thinking of something as a support to this universe? Everything is the aggregate of qualities; why should there be a hypothetical substance in which they should inhere? The idea of substance comes from the rapid interchange of qualities, not from something unchangeable which exists behind them. We see how wonderful some of these arguments are, and they appeal easily to the ordinary experience of humanity — in fact, not one in a million can think of anything other than phenomena. To the vast majority of men nature appears to be only a changing, whirling, combining, mingling mass of change. Few of us ever have a glimpse of the calm sea behind. For us it is always lashed into waves; this universe appears to us only as a tossing mass of waves. Thus we find these two opinions. One is that there is something behind both body and mind which is an unchangeable and immovable substance; and the other is that there is no such thing as immovability or unchangeability in the universe; it is all change and nothing but change. The solution of this difference comes in the next step of thought, namely, the non-dualistic.

It says that the dualists are right in finding something behind all, as a background which does not change; we cannot conceive change without there being something unchangeable. We can only conceive of anything that is changeable, by knowing something which is less changeable, and this also must appear more changeable in comparison with something else which is less changeable, and so on and on, until we are bound to admit that there must be something which never changes at all. The whole of this manifestation must have been in a state of non-manifestation, calm and silent, being the balance of opposing forces, so to say, when no force operated, because force acts when a disturbance of the equilibrium comes in. The universe is ever hurrying on to return to that state of equilibrium again. If we are certain of any fact whatsoever, we are certain of this. When the dualists claim that there is a something which does not change, they are perfectly right, but their analysis that it is an underlying something which is neither the body nor the mind, a something separate from both, is wrong. So far as the Buddhists say that the whole universe is a mass of change, they are perfectly right; so long as I am separate from the universe, so long as I stand back and look at something before me, so long as there are two things — the looker-on and the thing looked upon — it will appear always that the universe is one of change, continuously changing all the time. But the reality is that there is both change and changelessness in this universe. It is not that the soul and the mind and the body are three separate existences, for this organism made of these three is really one. It is the same thing which appears as the body, as the mind, and as the thing beyond mind and body, but it is not at the same time all these. He who sees the body does not see the mind even, he who sees the mind does not see that which he calls the soul, and he who sees the soul – for him the body and mind have vanished. He who sees only motion never sees absolute calm, and he who sees absolute calm – for him motion has vanished. A rope is taken for a snake. He who sees the rope as the snake, for him the rope has vanished, and when the delusion ceases and he looks at the rope, the snake has vanished.

There is then but one all-comprehending existence, and that one appears as manifold. This Self or Soul or Substance is all that exists in the universe. That Self or Substance or Soul is, in the language of non-dualism, the Brahman appearing to be manifold by the interposition of name and form. Look at the waves in the sea. Not one wave is really different from the sea, but what makes the wave apparently different? Name and form; the form of the wave and the name which we give to it, "wave". This is what makes it different from the sea. When name and form go, it is the same sea. Who can make any real difference between the wave and the sea? So this whole universe is that one Unit Existence; name and form have created all these various differences. As when the sun shines upon millions of globules of water, upon each particle is seen a most perfect representation of the sun, so the one Soul, the one Self, the one Existence of the universe, being reflected on all these numerous globules of varying names and forms, appears to be various. But it is in reality only one. There is no "I" nor "you"; it is all one. It is either all "I" or all "you". This idea of duality, calf two, is entirely false, and the whole universe, as we ordinarily know it, is the result of this false knowledge. When discrimination comes and man finds there are not two but one, he finds that he is himself this universe. "It is I who am this universe as it now exists, a continuous mass of change. It is I who am beyond all changes, beyond all qualities, the eternally perfect, the eternally blessed."

There is, therefore, but one Atman, one Self, eternally pure, eternally perfect, unchangeable, unchanged; it has never changed; and all these various changes in the universe are but appearances in that one Self.

Upon it name and form have painted all these dreams; it is the form that makes the wave different from the sea. Suppose the wave subsides, will the form remain? No, it will vanish. The existence of the wave was entirely dependent upon the existence of the sea, but the existence of the sea was not at all dependent upon the existence of the wave. The form remains so long as the wave remains, but as soon as the wave leaves it, it vanishes, it cannot remain. This name and form is the outcome of what is called Maya. It is this Maya that is making individuals, making one appear different from another. Yet it has no existence. Maya cannot be said to exist. Form cannot be said to exist, because it depends upon the existence of another thing. It cannot be said as not to exist, seeing that it makes all this difference. According to the Advaita philosophy, then, this Maya or ignorance — or name and form, or, as it has been called in Europe, "time, space, and causality" — is out of this one Infinite Existence showing us the manifoldness of the universe; in substance, this universe is one. So long as any one thinks that there are two ultimate realities, he is mistaken. When he has come to know that there is but one, he is right. This is what is being proved to us every day, on the physical plane, on the mental plane, and also on the spiritual plane. Today it has been demonstrated that you and I, the sun, the moon, and the stars are but the different names of different spots in the same ocean of matter, and that this matter is continuously changing in its configuration. This particle of energy that was in the sun several months ago may be in the human being now; tomorrow it may be in an animal, the day after tomorrow it may be in a plant. It is ever coming and going. It is all one unbroken, infinite mass of matter, only differentiated by names and forms. One point is called the sun; another, the moon; another, the stars; another, man; another, animal; another, plant; and so on. And all these names are fictitious; they have no reality, because the whole is a continuously changing mass of matter. This very same universe, from another standpoint, is an ocean of thought, where each one of us is a point called a particular mind. You are a mind, I am a mind, everyone is a mind; and the very same universe viewed from the standpoint of knowledge, when the eyes have been cleared of delusions, when the mind has become pure, appears to be the unbroken Absolute Being, the ever pure, the unchangeable, the immortal.

What then becomes of all this threefold eschatology of the dualist, that when a man dies he goes to heaven, or goes to this or that sphere, and that the wicked persons become ghosts, and become animals, and so forth? None comes and none goes, says the non-dualist. How can you come and go? You are infinite; where is the place for you to go? In a certain school a number of little children were being examined. The examiner had foolishly put all sorts of difficult questions to the little children. Among others there was this question: "Why does not the earth fall ?" His intention was to bring out the idea of gravitation or some other intricate scientific truth from these children. Most of them could not even understand the question, and so they gave all sorts of wrong answers. But one bright little girl answered it with another question: "Where shall it fall?" The very question of the examiner was nonsense on the face of it. There is no up and down in the universe; the idea is only relative. So it is with regard to the soul; the very question of birth and death in regard to it is utter nonsense. Who goes and who comes? Where are you not? Where is the heaven that you are not in already? Omnipresent is the Self of man. Where is it to go? Where is it not to go? It is everywhere. So all this childish dream and puerile illusion of birth and death, of heavens and higher heavens and lower worlds, all vanish immediately for the perfect. For the nearly perfect it vanishes after showing them the several scenes up to Brahmaloka. It continues for the ignorant.

How is it that the whole world believes in going to heaven, and in dying and being born? I am studying a book, page after page is being read and turned over. Another page comes and is turned over. Who changes? Who comes and goes? Not I, but the book. This whole nature is a book before the soul, chapter after chapter is being read and turned over, and every now and then a scene opens. That is read and turned over. A fresh one comes, but the soul is ever the same — eternal. It is nature that is changing, not the soul of man. This never changes. Birth and death are in nature, not in you.

Yet the ignorant are deluded; just as we under delusion think that the sun is moving and not the earth, in exactly the same way we think that we are dying, and not nature. These are all, therefore, hallucinations. Just as it is a hallucination when we think that the fields are moving and not the railway train, exactly in the same manner is the hallucination of birth and death. When men are in a certain frame of mind, they see this very existence as the earth, as the sun, the moon, the stars; and all those who are in the same state of mind see the same things. Between you and me there may be millions of beings on different planes of existence. They will never see us, nor we them; we only see those who are in the same state of mind and on the same plane with us. Those musical instruments respond which have the same attunement of vibration, as it were; if the state of vibration, which they call "man-vibration", should be changed, no longer would men be seen here; the whole "man-universe" would vanish, and instead of that, other scenery would come before us, perhaps gods and the god-universe, or perhaps, for the wicked man, devils and the diabolic world; but all would be only different views of the one universe. It is this universe which, from the human plane, is seen as the earth, the sun, the moon, the stars, and all such things – it is this very universe which, seen from the plane of wickedness, appears as a place of punishment. And this very universe is seen as heaven by those who want to see it as heaven. Those who have been dreaming of going to a God who is sitting on a throne, and of standing there praising Him all their lives, when they die, will simply see a vision of what they have in their minds; this very universe will simply change into a vast heaven, with all sorts of winged beings flying about and a God sitting on a throne. These heavens are all of man's own making. So what the dualist says is true, says the Advaitin, but it is all simply of his own making. These spheres and devils and gods and reincarnations and transmigrations are all mythology; so also is this human life. The great mistake that men always make is to think that this life alone is true. They understand it well enough when other things are called mythologies, but are never willing to admit the same of their own position. The whole thing as it appears is mere mythology, and the greatest of all lies is that we are bodies, which we never were nor even can be. It is the greatest of all lies that we are mere men; we are the God of the universe. In worshipping God we have been always worshipping our own hidden Self. The worst lie that you ever tell yourself is that you were born a sinner or a wicked man. He alone is a sinner who sees a sinner in another man. Suppose there is a baby here, and you place a bag of gold on the table. Suppose a robber comes and takes the gold away. To the baby it is all the same; because there is no robber inside, there is no robber outside. To sinners and vile men, there is vileness outside, but not to good men. So the wicked see this universe as a hell, and the partially good see it as heaven, while the perfect beings realise it as God Himself. Then alone the veil falls from the eyes, and the man, purified and cleansed, finds his whole vision changed. The bad dreams that have been torturing him for millions of years, all vanish, and he who was thinking of himself either as a man, or a god, or a demon, he who was thinking of himself as living in low places, in high places, on earth, in heaven, and so on, finds that he is really omnipresent; that all time is in him, and that he is not in time; that all the heavens are in him, that he is not in any heaven; and that all the gods that man ever worshipped are in him, and that he is not in any one of those gods. He was the manufacturer of gods and demons, of men and plants and animals and stones, and the real nature of man now stands unfolded to him as being higher than heaven, more perfect than this universe of ours, more infinite than infinite time, more omnipresent than the omnipresent ether. Thus alone man becomes fearless, and becomes free. Then all delusions cease, all miseries vanish, all fears come to an end for ever. Birth goes away and with it death; pains fly, and with them fly away pleasures; earths vanish, and with them vanish heavens; bodies vanish, and with them vanishes the mind also. For that man disappears the whole universe, as it were. This searching, moving, continuous struggle of forces stops for ever, and that which was manifesting itself as force and matter, as struggles of nature, as nature itself, as heavens and earths and plants and animals and men and angels, all that becomes transfigured into one infinite, unbreakable, unchangeable existence, and the knowing man finds that he is one with that existence. "Even as clouds of various colours come before the sky, remain there for a second and then vanish away," even so before this soul are all these visions coming, of earths and heavens, of the moon and the gods, of pleasures and pains; but they all pass away leaving the one infinite, blue, unchangeable sky. The sky never changes; it is the clouds that change. It is a mistake to think that the sky is changed. It is a mistake to think that we are impure, that we are limited, that we are separate. The real man is the one Unit Existence.

Two questions now arise. The first is: "Is it possible to realise this? So far it is doctrine, philosophy, but is it possible to realise it?" It is. There are men still living in this world for whom delusion has vanished for ever. Do they immediately die after such realisation? Not so soon as we should think. Two wheels joined by one pole are running together. If I get hold of one of the wheels and, with an axe, cut the pole asunder, the wheel which I have got hold of stops, but upon the other wheel is its past momentum, so it runs on a little arid then falls down. This pure and perfect being, the soul, is one wheel, and this external hallucination of body and mind is the other wheel, joined together by the pole of work, of Karma. Knowledge is the axe which will sever the bond between the two, and the wheel of the soul will stop — stop thinking that it is coming and going, living and dying, stop thinking that it is nature and has wants and desires, and will find that it is perfect, desireless. But upon the other wheel, that of the body and mind, will be the momentum of past acts; so it will live for some time, until that momentum of past work is exhausted, until that momentum is worked away, and then the body and mind fall, and the soul becomes free. No more is there any going to heaven and coming back, not even any going to the Brahmaloka, or to any of the highest of the spheres, for where is he to come from, or to go to? The man who has in this life attained to this state, for whom, for a minute at least, the ordinary vision of the world has changed and the reality has been apparent, he is called the "Living Free". This is the goal of the Vedantin, to attain freedom while living.

Once in Western India I was travelling in the desert country on the coast of the Indian Ocean. For days and days I used to travel on foot through the desert, but it was to my surprise that I saw every day beautiful lakes, with trees all round them, and the shadows of the trees upside down and vibrating there. "How wonderful it looks and they call this a desert country!" I said to myself. Nearly a month I travelled, seeing these wonderful lakes and trees and plants. One day I was very thirsty and wanted to have a drink of water, so I started to go to one of these clear, beautiful lakes, and as I approached, it vanished. And with a flash it came to my brain, "This is the mirage about which I have read all my life," and with that came also the idea that throughout the whole of this month, every day, I had been seeing the mirage and did not know it. The next morning I began my march. There was again the lake, but with it came also the idea that it was the mirage and not a true lake. So is it with this universe. We are all travelling in this mirage of the world day after day, month after month, year after year, not knowing that it is a mirage. One day it will break up, but it will come back again; the body has to remain under the power of past Karma, and so the mirage will come back. This world will come back upon us so long as we are bound by Karma: men, women, animals, plants, our attachments and duties, all will come back to us, but not with the same power. Under the influence of the new knowledge the strength of Karma will be broken, its poison will be lost. It becomes transformed, for along with it there comes the idea that we know it now, that the sharp distinction between the reality and the mirage has been known.

This world will not then be the same world as before. There is, however, a danger here. We see in every country people taking up this philosophy and saying, "I am beyond all virtue and vice; so I am not bound by any moral laws; I may do anything I like." You may find many fools in this country at the present time, saying, "I am not bound; I am God Himself; let me do anything I like." This is not right, although it is true that the soul is beyond all laws, physical, mental, or moral. Within law is bondage; beyond law is freedom. It is also true that freedom is of the nature of the soul, it is its birthright: that real freedom of the soul shines through veils of matter in the form of the apparent freedom of man. Every moment of your life you feel that you are free. We cannot live, talk, or breathe for a moment without feeling that we are free; but, at the same time, a little thought shows us that we are like machines and not free. What is true then? Is this idea of freedom a delusion? One party holds that the idea of freedom is a delusion; another says that the idea of bondage is a delusion. How does this happen? Man is really free, the real man cannot but be free. It is when he comes into the world of Maya, into name and form, that he becomes bound. Free will is a misnomer. Will can never be free. How can it be? It is only when the real man has become bound that his will comes into existence, and not before. The will of man is bound, but that which is the foundation of that will is eternally free. So, even in the state of bondage which we call human life or god-life, on earth or in heaven, there yet remains to us that recollection of the freedom which is ours by divine right. And consciously or unconsciously we are all struggling towards it. When a man has attained his own freedom, how can he be bound by any law? No law in this universe can bind him, for this universe itself is his.

He is the whole universe. Either say he is the whole universe or say that to him there is no universe. How can he have then all these little ideas about sex and about country? How can he say, I am a man, I am a woman I am a child? Are they not lies? He knows that they are. How can he say that these are man's rights, and these others are woman's rights? Nobody has rights; nobody separately exists. There is neither man nor woman; the soul is sexless, eternally pure. It is a lie to say that I am a man or a woman, or to say that I belong to this country or that. All the world is my country, the whole universe is mine, because I have clothed myself with it as my body. Yet we see that there are people in this world who are ready to assert these doctrines, and at the same time do things which we should call filthy; and if we ask them why they do so, they tell us that it is our delusion and that they can do nothing wrong. What is the test by which they are to be judged? The test is here.

Though evil and good are both conditioned manifestations of the soul, yet evil is the most external coating, and good is the nearer coating of the real man, the Self. And unless a man cuts through the layer of evil he cannot reach the layer of good, and unless he has passed through both the layers of good and evil he cannot reach the Self. He who reaches the Self, what remains attached to him? A little Karma, a little bit of the momentum of past life, but it is all good momentum. Until the bad momentum is entirely worked out and past impurities are entirely burnt, it is impossible for any man to see and realise truth. So, what is left attached to the man who has reached the Self and seen the truth is the remnant of the good impressions of past life, the good momentum. Even if he lives in the body and works incessantly, he works only to do good; his lips speak only benediction to all; his hands do only good works; his mind can only think good thoughts; his presence is a blessing wherever he goes. He is himself a living blessing. Such a man will, by his very presence, change even the most wicked persons into saints. Even if he does not speak, his very presence will be a blessing to mankind. Can such men do any evil; can they do wicked deeds? There is, you must remember, all the difference of pole to pole between realisation and mere talking. Any fool can talk. Even parrots talk. Talking is one thing, and realising is another. Philosophies, and doctrines, and arguments, and books, and theories, and churches, and sects, and all these things are good in their own way; but when that realisation comes, these things drop away. For instance, maps are good, but when you see the country itself, and look again at the maps, what a great difference you find! So those that have realised truth do not require the ratiocinations of logic and all other gymnastics of the intellect to make them understand the truth; it is to them the life of their lives, concretised, made more than tangible. It is, as the sages of the Vedanta say, "even as a fruit in your hand"; you can stand up and say, it is here. So those that have realised the truth will stand up and say, "Here is the Self". You may argue with them by the year, but they will smile at you; they will regard it all as child's prattle; they will let the child prattle on. They have realised the truth and are full. Suppose you have seen a country, and another man comes to you and tries to argue with you that that country never existed, he may go on arguing indefinitely, but your only attitude of mind towards him must be to hold that the man is fit for a lunatic asylum.

So the man of realisation says, "All this talk in the world about its little religions is but prattle; realisation is the soul, the very essence of religion." Religion can be realised. Are you ready? Do you want it? You will get the realisation if you do, and then you will be truly religious. Until you have attained realisation there is no difference between you and atheists. The atheists are sincere, but the man who says that he believes in religion and never attempts to realise it is not sincere.

The next question is to know what comes after realisation. Suppose we have realised this oneness of the universe, that we are that one Infinite Being, and suppose we have realised that this Self is the only Existence and that it is the same Self which is manifesting in all these various phenomenal forms, what becomes of us after that? Shall we become inactive, get into a corner and sit down there and die away? "What good will it do to the world?" That old question! In the first place, why should it do good to the world? Is there any reason why it should? What right has any one to ask the question, "What good will it do to the world?" What is meant by that? A baby likes candies. Suppose you are conducting investigations in connection with some subject of electricity and the baby asks you, "Does it buy candies?" "No" you answer. "Then what good will it do?" says the baby. So men stand up and say, "What good will this do to the world; will it give us money?" "No." "Then what good is there in it?" That is what men mean by doing good to the world. Yet religious realisation does all the good to the world. People are afraid that when they attain to it, when they realise that there is but one, the fountains of love will be dried up, that everything in life will go away, and that all they love will vanish for them, as it were, in this life and in the life to come. People never stop to think that those who bestowed the least thought on their own individualities have been the greatest workers in the world. Then alone a man loves when he finds that the object of his love is not any low, little, mortal thing. Then alone a man loves when he finds that the object of his love is not a clod of earth, but it is the veritable God Himself. The wife will love the husband the more when she thinks that the husband is God

Himself. The husband will love the wife the more when he knows that the wife is God Himself. That mother will love the children more who thinks that the children are God Himself. That man will love his greatest enemy who knows that that very enemy is God Himself. That man will love a holy man who knows that the holy man is God Himself, and that very man will also love the unholiest of men because he knows the background of that unholiest of men is even He, the Lord. Such a man becomes a world-mover for whom his little self is dead and God stands in its place. The whole universe will become transfigured to him. That which is painful and miserable will all vanish; struggles will all depart and go. Instead of being a prison-house, where we every day struggle and fight and compete for a morsel of bread, this universe will then be to us a playground. Beautiful will be this universe then! Such a man alone has the right to stand up and say, "How beautiful is this world!" He alone has the right to say that it is all good. This will be the great good to the world resulting from such realisation, that instead of this world going on with all its friction and clashing, if all mankind today realise only a bit of that great truth, the aspect of the whole world will be changed, and, in place of fighting and quarrelling, there would be a reign of peace. This indecent and brutal hurry which forces us to go ahead of every one else will then vanish from the world. With it will vanish all struggle, with it will vanish all hate, with it will vanish all jealousy, and all evil will vanish away for ever. Gods will live then upon this earth. This very earth will then become heaven, and what evil can there be when gods are playing with gods, when gods are working with gods, and gods are loving gods? That is the great utility of divine realisation. Everything that you see in society will be changed and transfigured then. No more will you think of man as evil; and that is the first great gain. No more will you stand up and sneeringly cast a glance at a poor man or woman who has made a mistake. No more, ladies, will you look down with contempt upon the poor woman who walks the street in the night, because you will see even there God Himself. No more will you think of jealousy and punishments. They will all vanish; and love, the great ideal of love, will be so powerful that no whip and cord will be necessary to guide mankind aright.

If one millionth part of the men and women who live in this world simply sit down and for a few minutes say, "You are all God, O ye men and O ye animals and living beings, you are all the manifestations of the one living Deity!" the whole world will be changed in half an hour. Instead of throwing tremendous bomb-shells of hatred into every corner, instead of projecting currents of jealousy and of evil thought, in every country people will think that it is all He. He is all that you see and feel. How can you see evil until there is evil in you? How can you see the thief, unless he is there, sitting in the heart of your heart? How can you see the murderer until you are yourself the murderer? Be good, and evil will vanish for you. The whole universe will thus be changed. This is the greatest gain to society. This is the great gain to the human organism. These thoughts were thought out, worked out amongst individuals in ancient times in India. For various reasons, such as the exclusiveness of the teachers and foreign conquest, those thoughts were not allowed to spread. Yet they are grand truths; and wherever they have been working, man has become divine. My whole life has been changed by the touch of one of these divine men, about whom I am going to speak to you next Sunday; and the time is coming when these thoughts will be cast abroad over the whole world. Instead of living in monasteries, instead of being confined to books of philosophy to be studied only by the learned, instead of being the exclusive possession of sects and of a few of the learned, they will all be sown broadcast over the whole world, so that they may become the common property of the saint and the sinner, of men and women and children, of the learned and of the ignorant. They will then permeate the atmosphere of the world, and the very air that we breathe will say with every one of its pulsations, "Thou art That". And the whole universe with its myriads of suns and moons, through everything that speaks, with one voice will say, "Thou art That".

❑❑❑